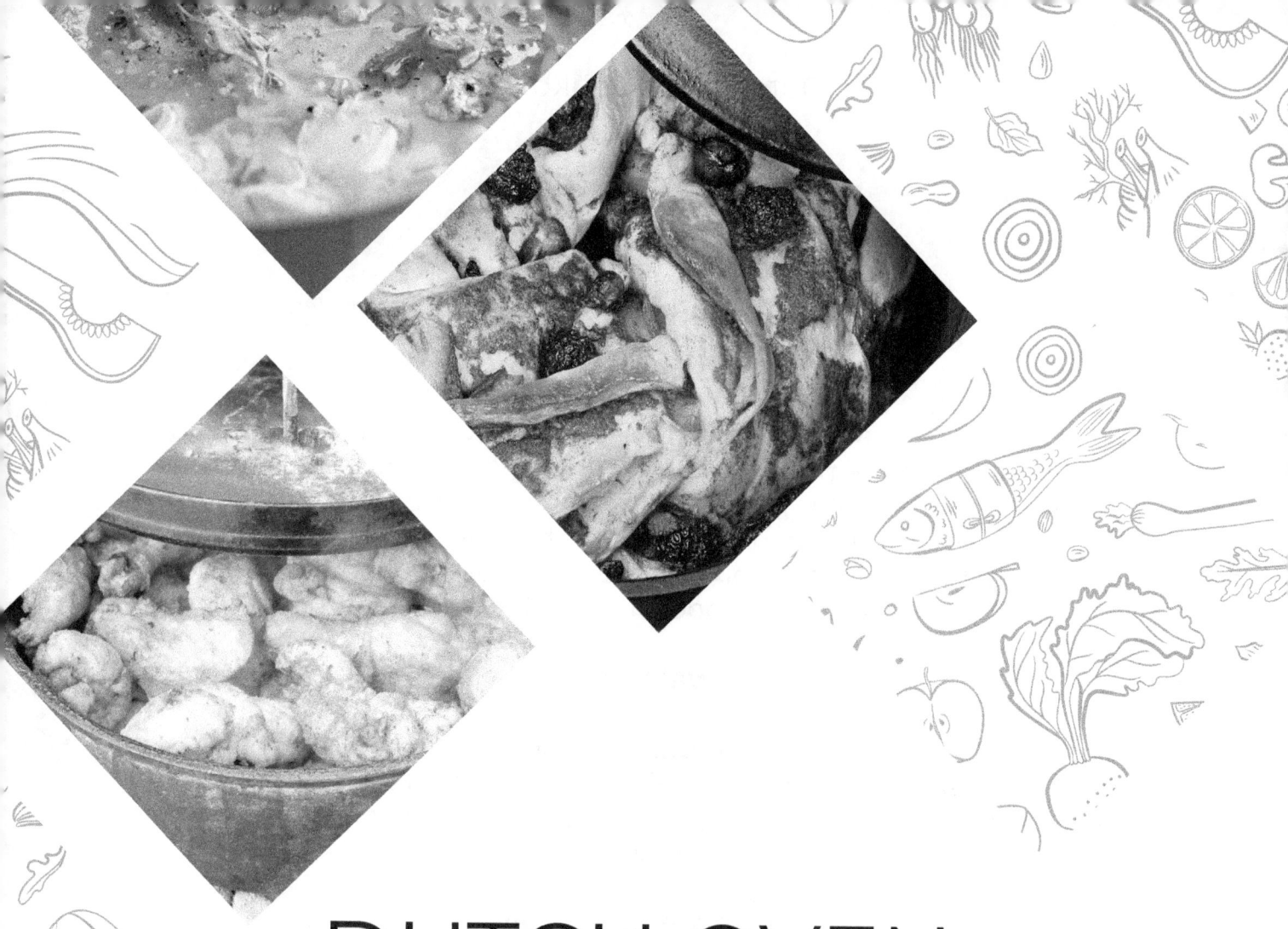

DUTCH OVEN
Cookbook

200 Foolproof 5-Ingredient Recipes. Quick and Easy One Pot Flavorful Meals for Everyday Cooking

Vivian Bayne

Copyright - 2020 - All rights reserved.

The content contained within this book may not be reproduced, duplicated or transmitted without direct written permission from the author or the publisher. Under no circumstances will any blame or legal responsibility be held against the publisher, or author, for any damages, reparation, or monetary loss due to the information contained within this book. Either directly or indirectly.

Legal Notice:

This book is copyright protected. This book is only for personal use. You cannot amend, distribute, sell, use, quote or paraphrase any part, or the content within this book, without the consent of the author or publisher.

Disclaimer Notice:

Please note the information contained within this document is for educational and entertainment purposes only. All effort has been executed to present accurate, up to date, and reliable, complete information. No warranties of any kind are declared or implied. Readers acknowledge that the author is not engaging in the rendering of legal, financial, medical or professional advice. The content within this book has been derived from various sources. Please consult a licensed professional before attempting any techniques outlined in this book.

By reading this document, the reader agrees that under no circumstances is the author responsible for any losses, direct or indirect, which are incurred as a result of the use of information contained within this document, including, but not limited to, - errors, omissions, or inaccuracies.

Dutch Oven Cookbook

TABLE OF CONTENTS

INTRODUCTION	5
BREAKFAST	13
POULTRY	22
BEEF	70
BREAD, ROLLS AND BISCUITS	92
DESSERT RECIPES	102
CONCLUSION	117

INDEX OF RECIPES AT THE END OF THE BOOK

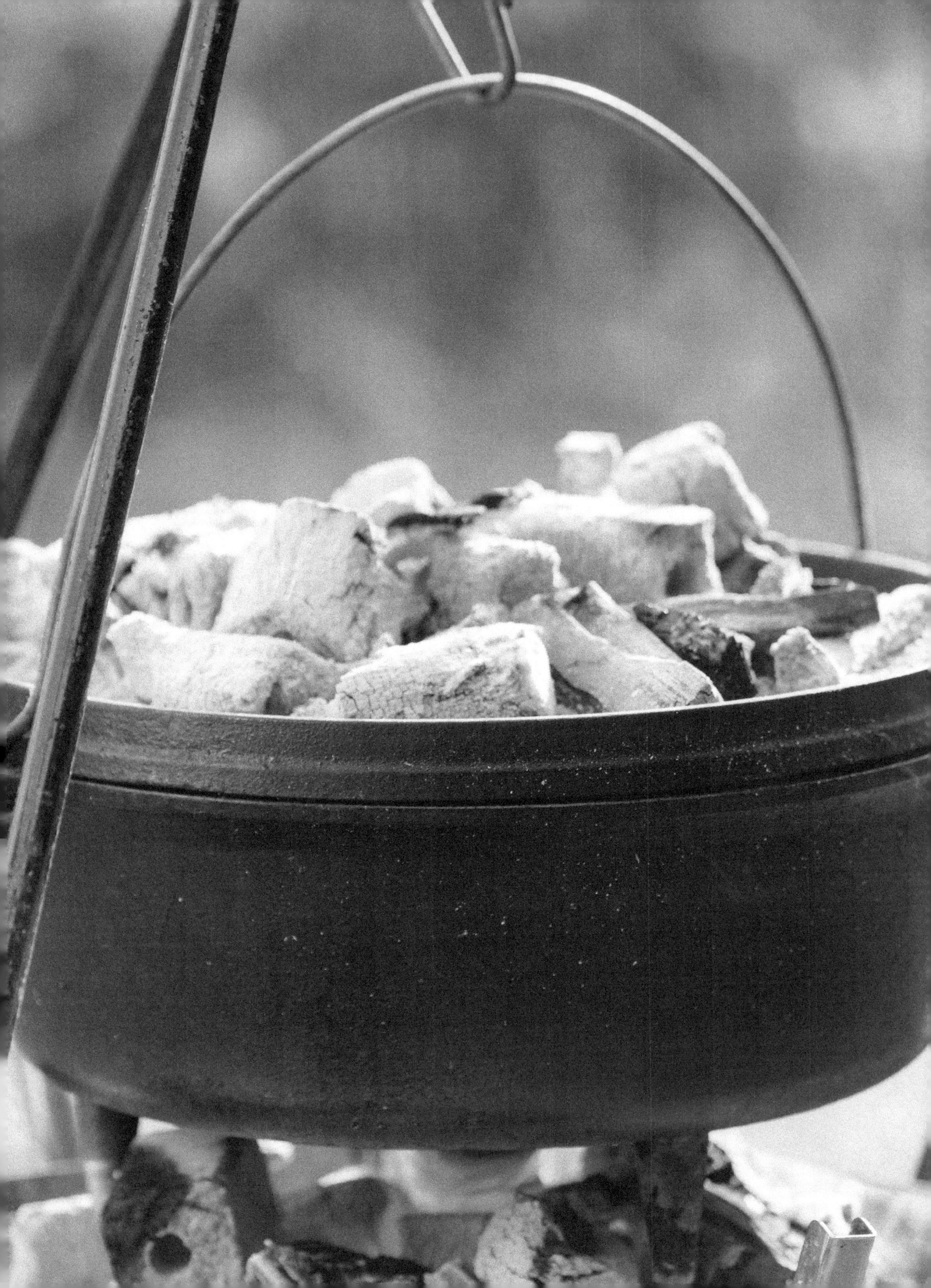

Dutch Oven Cookbook

INTRODUCTION

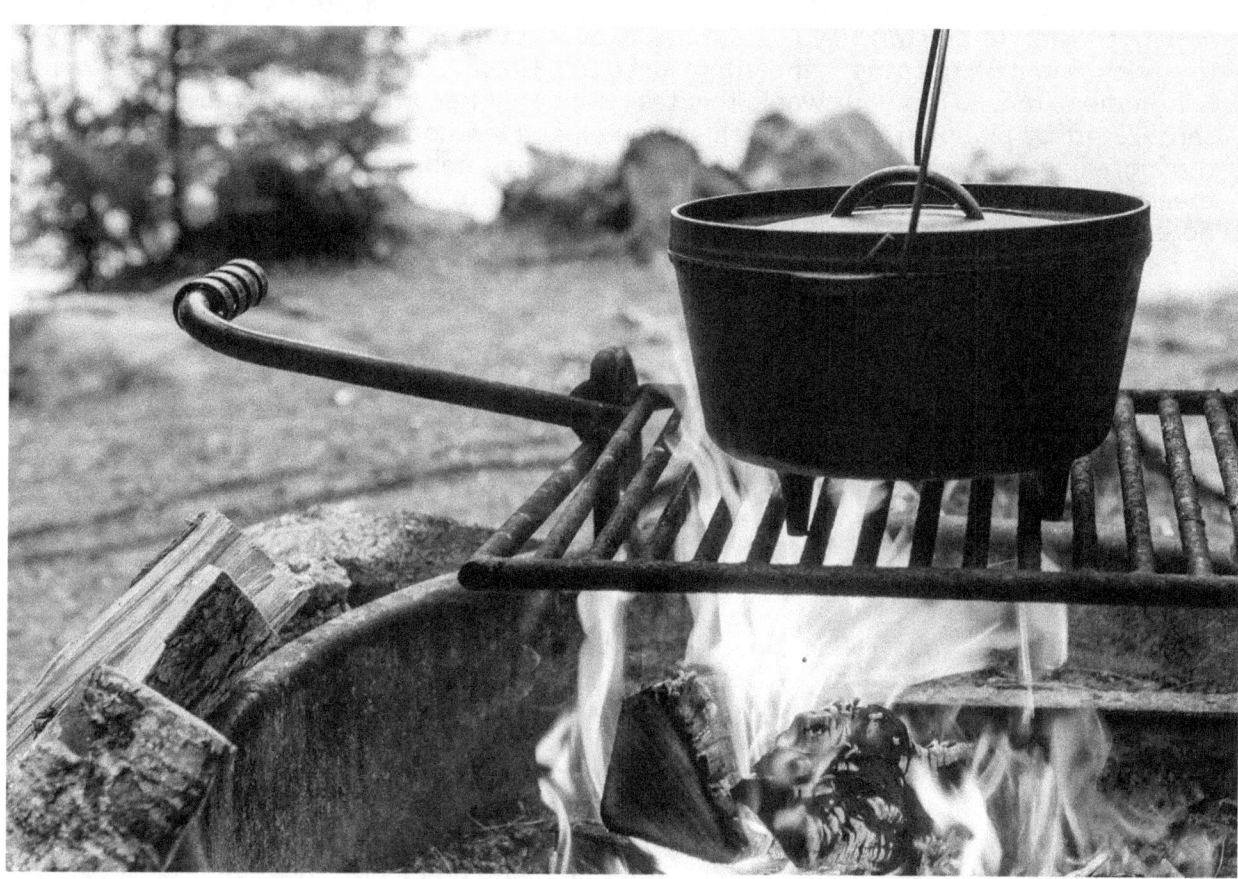

Cooking, for many, is an enjoyable and rewarding activity. For some, it is just the sheer pleasure of providing friends and family with a nourishing meal, while others see their culinary creations as a form of artistic expression. Unfortunately, our everyday lifestyles' hectic pace leaves little time for crafting and expression in the kitchen for many of us. Instead, we turn to prepackaged foods, less nutritious ingredients, and meals on the go. This is not a healthy way to live for either the body or the spirit.

Recently the trend in culinary styles has turned toward simplicity. There has been a focus on advanced preparation such as freezer meals or meal parties where friends and family get together to prepare a week or a month's worth of meals together at one time. The point here is to have wholesome foods in your life while still making time for the other people and things that are important to you. To further simplify the process, there has been an additional priority placed on using fewer ingredients, which leads to a savings of time, money, energy, and to the use of the freshest, most flavorful ingredients available.

SHOPPING FOR 5-INGREDIENT MEALS

One of the first areas of your life that 5-ingredient meals will make an improvement in is your budget! You will soon discover that you do not need to buy a lot of ingredients to create one delicious meal. Often, the exact opposite is true. Fewer ingredients mean that you can let each one shine on their own without overly complicating their flavor profiles. Here are a few tips to make shopping for your 5-ingredient lifestyle easier and more efficient.

First, start with a meal plan. As someone that tends to overcomplicate something as simple as a meal plan, I understand if you may initially bulk at this. Some have meal planning down to a science, but on the other hand, some just don't. However, when you incorporate several 5-ingredient meals into your week, this task suddenly becomes easier and makes more sense. Start by planning on one breakfast, one lunch, and one dinner. Now take a look at the ingredients that you are using for those three meals and compile a list of at least three meals that you can make using the same ingredients with few or no add-ons. Also, make a note of the staples you use in your home every week and see how you can effectively work them into 5-ingredient dishes. Items such as eggs, oil, milk, grains, and cheese are used in many 5-ingredient dishes.

Always choose the freshest ingredients available to you. The fresher your food is the more flavorful it will be. The only problem with this is that some foods perish quickly. This can make for multiple trips to the grocery store each week. To reduce the incidence of that, take advantage of produce at its seasonal peak of freshness and freeze it yourself. If instead, you feel like venturing into the world of naturally canned and preserved food, you should get my Best Seller book Canning and Preserving for Beginners - The Complete Guide to Can and Preserve any Food in Jars, with Easy and Tasty Recipes. Learn how to Preserve and Cook Veggies, Fruit, Meat, Poultry, Fish and More.

Even after freezing, you will find that these foods retain a freshness quality that just can't be found in conventional frozen foods from your grocer. Take advantage of "freebie" ingredients. Typically, with 5-ingredient meals, ingredients such as water and simple seasonings like salt and pepper are not included in the ingredients' grand total. Other spices may not be listed in a recipe because the goal is to reduce the number of ingredients that you need to buy and prepare. However, you should always take advantage of the spices available in your home and that you commonly use in your cooking. A little bit of your favorite spice can make the difference between something you find bland and a dish that you find exciting. Keep some basics in your pantry. When you do your grocery shopping, make sure that you are adequately stocked on the staples that you use in your family. Items such as grains, pasta, and beans are easy to prepare and can certainly be added into any meal to complement and add more substance to a meal if needed.

WHAT YOU NEED TO KNOW ABOUT DUTCH OVENS

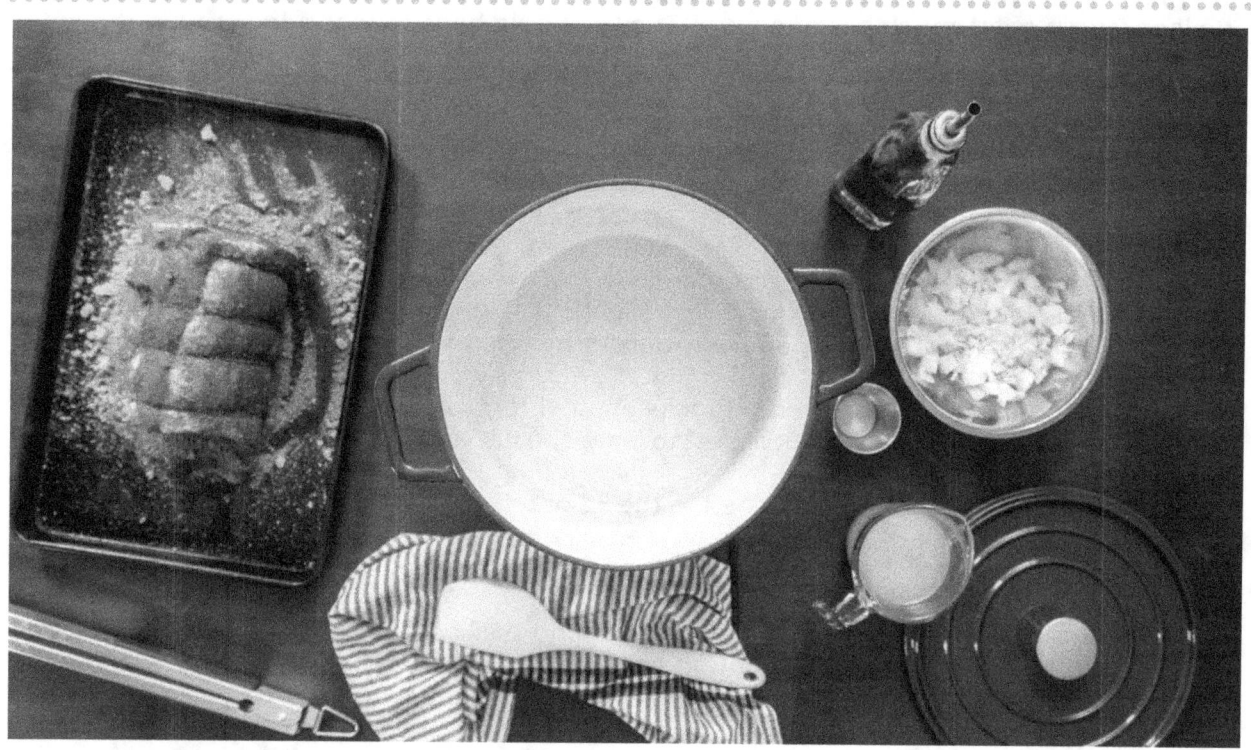

WHAT CAN THE DUTCH OVEN DO?
The Dutch oven is basically a heavy container pot with a tight-fitting lid.
This cast iron pot may look like an outdoor cooking appliance, but in reality, can also be a gift to home chefs around the world. In a Dutch oven, you can cook almost anything.
We're talking about one-pot meals, such as Alfredo pasta and tomato sauces, soups, sandwiches, biscuits, chili, beef stew, casserole, and the preparation of individual ingredients, such as sauces and garnishes.

You can even cut down on cooking time with a Dutch oven, because the pot can go straight into the oven from the stovetop without missing a beat, and you can put all of your ingredients in one bowl for many Dutch oven recipes.
Dutch ovens have been used for hundreds of years. Nothing will maintain a decent temperature better than the heavy metal in this monster bowl.
Let's discuss some of the things you need to know before we get started.

There are hundreds of Dutch oven variations available in the market, so it would be impossible for me to tell you which oven is for you.
Because each kind of oven is designed to cook in a different situation, I'm going to go over the various options, and you're going to have to decide what's best for you. When shopping for your oven, you should aim for one that is well-made. I would never compromise on quality when it comes to cooking!

Dutch Oven Cookbook

If you're looking for an outdoor Dutch oven, examine the bail handle. It should have a heavy gauge wire on the side of the oven and be firmly connected to shaped tangs. Avoid ovens that have riveted tabs.

Most of the oven handles lie in both directions against the side of the oven, but with close examination, you can find some with a handle that stands at an angle of 45 degrees on one leg. The handle on the lid should also be carefully examined. There should be a loop attached to both ends of the cover, and it should be hollow in the center for easy locking. Stay away from those with a sturdy shaped tab for a handle on the door.

An improper lid will be very difficult to grasp and handle, especially when using a lot of coal. The loop layout offers much better control. The lid should have a lip or ridge around the outer edge.

The lip prevents the coal from falling off the lid. You can use the ridge-less version, but it's hard to keep the coal on the lid, and if you're not careful to clean the ash from the lid every time you open the oven, you'll end up with ash and sand in your food.

Having a lip solves this issue practically. The lid can be removed with little difficulty, even if fully loaded with ash and coals.

The legs are another feature to examine carefully. While flat-bottomed ovens and four-legged ovens are available, the most common type has three legs. The legs are a must for outdoor cooking; they maintain the oven above ground's height providing ventilation for the coals below.

The flat-bottom oven can be placed on rocks or steel tent pegs with little risk of falling over. Murphy's law dictates though that it is best to leave the flat bottom ovens in the store or on the kitchen stove where they belong.

Finally, look for a second handle attached to the lid or top rim at the base of the oven.

Many ovens are available with a handle of the skillet type attached to the lid. This is a good idea in theory, but in fact, it seems that they are more in the way and don't provide adequate support.

These handles also get in the way during storage and packaging. It is essential to avoid fixed handles on the base of the oven, although I believe the theory behind these handles was to promote the placement of the oven in a deep fireplace.

Take a couple red bricks with you to the store and put them in an oven with this type of handle. Then try to raise the pot with the handle, and you'll see that the handle is useless. A loaded oven can be a real wrist-breaker, weighing 20 to 25 lbs.

The only exception is often a small tab on the oven's upper lip, which is about 1/2 to 1" deep and 2 to3" long. This tab makes it very easy to pour liquids from the oven, and its small size has never caused storage or packaging issues.

Many people immediately think "Cast Iron" when someone suggests a "Dutch Oven," but Dutch ovens can also be made of aluminum. An aluminum oven weighs just about 6.5 to 7 lbs., compared to about 18 lbs. for the cast-iron oven.

Each material has advantages and disadvantages. The most apparent benefit of aluminum is weight, 1 lb. lighter. Also, because aluminum does not rust, treatment is limited to essential soap and water cleaning.

Aluminum tends to heat quicker, taking less preheating time, but they do not hold the heat for long after removing from the coals. Because aluminum also reflects more heat than cast iron, it will take more coals to reach a set temperature and sustain it.

You will also see a more significant temperature variation on windy days with an aluminum Dutch Oven. Where weight is essential, it is possible to overcome most of the disadvantages of aluminum.

This type of temperature can be created if the oven is placed directly on the coals or when there are too many coals below the oven.

OTHER THINGS YOU MIGHT NEED

A reliable pair of leather gloves can save time around a fire and prove invaluable. A couple of

work style gloves are going to do that, but I suggest that you look for a fire and safety supply house or store that sells fireplace accessories and find a couple of fire handling gloves.
The extra protection and efficiency far outweigh the few extra dollars that fire handling gloves cost. You'll have to weigh the standard for yourself against the higher price.
You are going to need a shovel. The typical garden shovel will be enough. It will be used to heat and raise the coals to the oven from the fire pit. The handle's style and length are up to you. The long-handled shovels are great on hikes and canoe trips, but not practical for use with ovens. While the short "army" shovels are perfect for hiking and canoeing, they suffer from short handles, getting too close to the fire and risking burns. A pair of hot pot pliers is another object that will prove worth its weight in gold.

DUTCH OVEN TYPES

Camping: These Dutch ovens have three legs to keep the coals off, a wire bail handle, and a slightly concave, rimmed cover to place the coals or briquettes on top and bottom. It makes internal heat more consistent and allows the inside to act as an oven. Usually, these ovens were made of bare cast iron.
Cooking methods such as roasting, baking, stewing, frying, boiling, steaming, and many others are quickly done on the campfire with just one utensil, the Dutch oven.
These and many more are very possible and sometimes simpler than at home. With very few exceptions, you'll be able to duplicate home recipes with the Dutch oven on the campfire.
Modern: These Dutch ovens are designed to be used on the stove or in the oven and usually have a lipless top.

Like the unglazed ovens, many older types retained the handle, while others, like the enameled, had two handles of the ring. Traditional Dutch ovens consist of cast iron, cast aluminum, or ceramic.
Usually, there are two cooking methods used with the Modern Dutch oven. The first method places the food in the Dutch oven's center. In the second method, food is cooked in a second dish and then placed in the bottom of the Dutch oven on a trivet. The trivet's purpose is to lift the plate above the bottom of the oven to avoid burning.

SELECTING/BUYING A DUTCH OVEN

Camping Dutch ovens are usually bought from hardware stores or sporting goods shops. New Dutch ovens can be sold in supermarkets or in cooking supply shops for the stovetop or traditional oven.
Determine the size, style as well as form needed when buying a Dutch oven. The Dutch aluminum oven is popular with backpackers as it is lighter, rustproof and does not need to be seasoned.
If you choose an aluminum oven, be careful not to overheat the oven because this can permanently damage the pan. Many people prefer cast iron ovens because they heat more uniformly and remain hot longer. Typically, the cost is about the same.

Diameter	Weight	Capacity	Serving Capacity
8"	3 lbs.	2 quarts	2-4 people
10"	5.5 lbs.	4 quarts	4-6 people
12"	7.5 lbs.	6 quarts	6-10 people
14"	9.5 lbs.	8 quarts	10-12 people
16"	11 lbs.	10 quarts	13-15 people
18"	13 lbs.	12 quarts	16-18 people
20"	14.5 lb.	14 quarts	19-22 people

Dutch Oven Cookbook

Choose the Dutch oven that best suits your needs. Dutch ovens are also available in various sizes and use a size numbering system. The table below shows the various size, weight and capacity.

DUTCH OVEN TOOLS

There are plenty of Dutch oven gadgets designed to help you quickly use your oven while cooking outdoors. The long-handled hooked lid remover is one of the most useful tools.
Such devices promote the cooking of the outdoor Dutch oven. No special tools are needed when using a Dutch oven on a stovetop or in a conventional oven.

PREPARATION OF YOUR OVEN

For aluminum, washing well with soap and water is the only necessary pre-treatment. Many aluminum ovens are delivered with a protective covering that can be removed by quick washing. Cast-iron ovens will last a lifetime if properly cared for. I know several people who have Dutch ovens belonging to great-grandmothers, dating way back to the 1800s.
Although this book is geared towards Dutch ovens, any cast iron skillet, grid, etc. is subject to the treatment and care instructions. The secret of the long life of cast iron is no mystery at all. Constant and careful maintenance will keep the oven in operation for many years, starting with the day it is purchased. Both standard Dutch ovens are shipped with a protective coating that should be removed.

You will need to use steel wool and some elbow grease to scrub your new oven. Clean the oven thoroughly, dry with a towel, and let air dry. While it is drying, it would be a good time to preheat your kitchen oven to 350 degrees Farenheit.
When it appears dry, place the Dutch oven on the center rack with the lid ajar. Let the Dutch oven to warm slowly, so it's just barely too hot for bare hands to touch. This pre-heating removes any residual moisture and opens the metal pores.
 Now, add a thin layer of salt-free cooking oil using a clean cloth or, ideally a paper towel. You can use oils such as almond oil, olive oil or vegetable oil. Tallow or lard will also do, but these animal fats tend to break down during the storage times and are not recommended for typical Dutch ovens during campouts.

Make sure that the oil coats every inch of the oven, inside and outside, and place the oven with the lid ajar on the center rack. Bake at 350 degrees Farenheit for an hour or so. This baking transforms the oil into a metal protective coating.
Let the oven cool slowly after baking. When handling is safe, add another thin oil coating. Repeat the process of baking and cooling.
When it can be treated again, reapply a thin oil coating. Now let the oven cool down completely. This treatment requires three layers of butter, two poured on, and one added warmly. The oven is now ready to be used or stored.

This pre-treatment process is only necessary once unless rust forms or the coating becomes damaged in storage or use. Anything baked on the surface will turn black with age and darken. This darkening is a symbol of an oven that is well maintained and used. The pre-treatment coating forms a barrier between air moisture and the metal surface. It effectively stops the metal from rusting, and provides the inside of the oven with a non-stick coating. This coating is as non-adhesive as most of the commercially applied coatings when adequately maintained.

SEASONING

First things first. Thoroughly wash the Dutch oven with soap and water and remove the protective cover. After that, either put it in your house or place it on a camp stove large enough to support its weight and let it thoroughly dry.
When dry, preheat your regular oven to 450 or 500 degrees Farenheit. Slightly brush the inside and outside of your Dutch oven with grease while the oven is preheating.
There are many different types of grease that you can use, from bacon to olive oil. Crisco in a tin is what I use. Do not use the scent of butter either.

Dutch Oven Cookbook

When the oven is preheated, place loosely-greased Dutch oven in it and roast it for an hour. Remove the Dutch oven and let it cool. Don't turn off your oven.

The Dutch oven should now feel tacky. If it does, place it in the oven for another 30 minutes set for 300 to 350 degrees Farenheit. The process will take two hours.

Seasoning stops the iron from being absorbed into the cast iron and taint the way food tastes. Properly sealed pans have an easy to clean non-stick finish. With age and use, pans that are adequately cared for get better and better.

There are two methods to season your Dutch oven. One is to thoroughly clean and dry and then apply half of the oil. Then heat until the oil swirls to cover all the inside surfaces. Dispose of used oil and substitute with fresh oil.

SEASONING YOUR DUTCH OVEN AGAIN

Suppose you did the unthinkable and left your Dutch oven all winter in the rain, and it rusted out, or you put it away, and the grease turned rancid.

You have two choices. You can buy a new oven, or you can clean it up. It's effortless to tell if your oven has become rancid, remove the lid and cover your nose.

It's rancid if you start gagging! You can also tell from the pot's hue; it turns a yellow-orange and looks gummy. Fill the oven with water; add a cup of vinegar and cook for half an hour.

Sprinkle the bath, clean and re-season your oven. You can remove mile rust in several ways. Use a steel wool pad first, and if it doesn't work, soak the oven. As a last resort, add a cup of apple cider vinegar and ample water and cover your oven with hay.

You need to be patient and wait with these soaking methods. Sandblasting is definitely a last resort. When using this approach, you have to be careful. Determine what sandblasting method to use. I was told that sand would take away the cast iron in the process, but glass beads will not. I made some calls, and the places where car bodywork is done also cleaned Dutch Ovens!

A Few DON'Ts

Do not allow cast iron to sit in water or let water stand in or on it. In spite of a durable coating, it will rust.

Never use the cast iron soap. The soap will get into the metal pores, and it won't come out very quickly, but it will come back to taint your next meal. When soap is used unintentionally, the pre-treatment process should be extended to the oven, including removal of the present coating.

Do not put an empty cast iron pan, or oven over a fire. It can be better handled by aluminum and many other metals, but cast iron can crack or warp and destroy this.

Do not heat cast iron in a hurry. You will end up with burnt food or an oven or pan that is fried. Never put cold liquid in a pan or oven of scorching cast iron. They're going to crack

COOKING TIPS

Dutch oven cooking can be done using a conventional oven or cooking top, a camp stove, a wood fire or charcoal briquettes on the back porch,

Choose the best source of heat for your purposes. The wood fire and heat sources for briquets are the most challenging to use as heat control is difficult.

The Dutch cast iron oven retains the heat and uniformly cooks food. You have a more regulated heat source when using your conventional oven, stovetop, or a camp stove.

A Dutch oven allows the cooking time to be decreased because it retains the heat longer. It takes less space to cook food.

Dutch Oven Cookbook

FIREWOOD COOKING

Wood campfires when you have a bank of hot coals are good for cooking. Prepare a sufficiently large fire. Cover the top and bottom of the oven with enough coals.

Partially burned and burning material smoke is hard to handle and will not maintain the necessary heat to thoroughly cook the food. Build a large coal bank and dig a shallow pit with a long-handled shovel. Shovel a sheet of coals onto the field. Put the oven in the coals and top the oven with a layer of coals and cover with soil. Be careful not to dislodge the lid. When the food is cooked scrape off the dirt and coals.

Coals are usually hot, and only experience can determine how hot the coals are.

Cooking With Briquettes

Light the briquettes, and let them get hot and grey. The oven's size will determine the number of necessary briquettes.

The general rule of thumb is to remember your Dutch oven's size. The number of coals on top of the oven is equal to the size. For the bottom, you are going to use half that number of briquettes.

Temperature

You can see that every briquette of charcoal is worth around 25 degrees Fahrenheit. Twenty coals will offer about 500 degrees.

Food checking

Food can be checked by lifting the whole Dutch Oven out and away from the fire or coals. Move the coals or briquettes out, and use the handle to lift the lid straight up and down.

Remove the lid carefully and put it on a clean surface. Use a folded piece of paper towel to clean around the edge where the cover and the oven meet.

Chop vegetables and meat and add moisture if needed to see if they are cooked. Attempt to remove the lid quickly before losing too much heat. Change the coals to remove some of the coals from the top or bottom of the oven if they are too dry.

If the food is slow to cook, add more hot coals. Replace the oven to the heat source and cook until the meal is finished.

Meat

It's beautiful to serve meats in a Dutch oven. They have a taste that you will never replicate using any other form of cooking.

Although the flavor is always excellent, it is difficult for some Dutch oven users to produce visually appealing meat from the steamy oven.

The trick is simple: irrespective of the spices and flavors you use on any meat or poultry, brown the meat first. Add enough butter, bacon or fat in the hot oven to brown the meat to make a good oil cover on the bottom, heat the oven, then place the meat in the oven and sear or brown well.

This will lock in natural juices and provide the texture and color more typical of grilled or fried meats.

Once the meat has browned well on all sides, remove any residual fat droppings, add any seasonings you want, put on the lid and cook for 30 to 35 minutes for one lb. of beef or lamb, and for 25 to 30 minutes for one lb. of poultry.

Vegetables

Garden vegetables are perfect additions to any Dutch oven meal. Many Dutch oven vegetables are prepared in some sauce, but they may be steamed or cooked on a conventional stove.

However, if you choose to roast or bake Dutch oven vegetables, they can cook around three minutes per inch of the oven's diameter.

A squash-filled 10-inch oven will cook for about 30 minutes; 36 minutes in the 12-inch oven. Cook vegetables in sauces, such as new peas and potatoes in white sauce, broccoli in cheese sauce or sour cream potatoes. They should be brought to a fast boil, water discarded, sauces added and boiled at the appropriate time for other vegetables.

Dutch Oven Cookbook

BREAKFAST

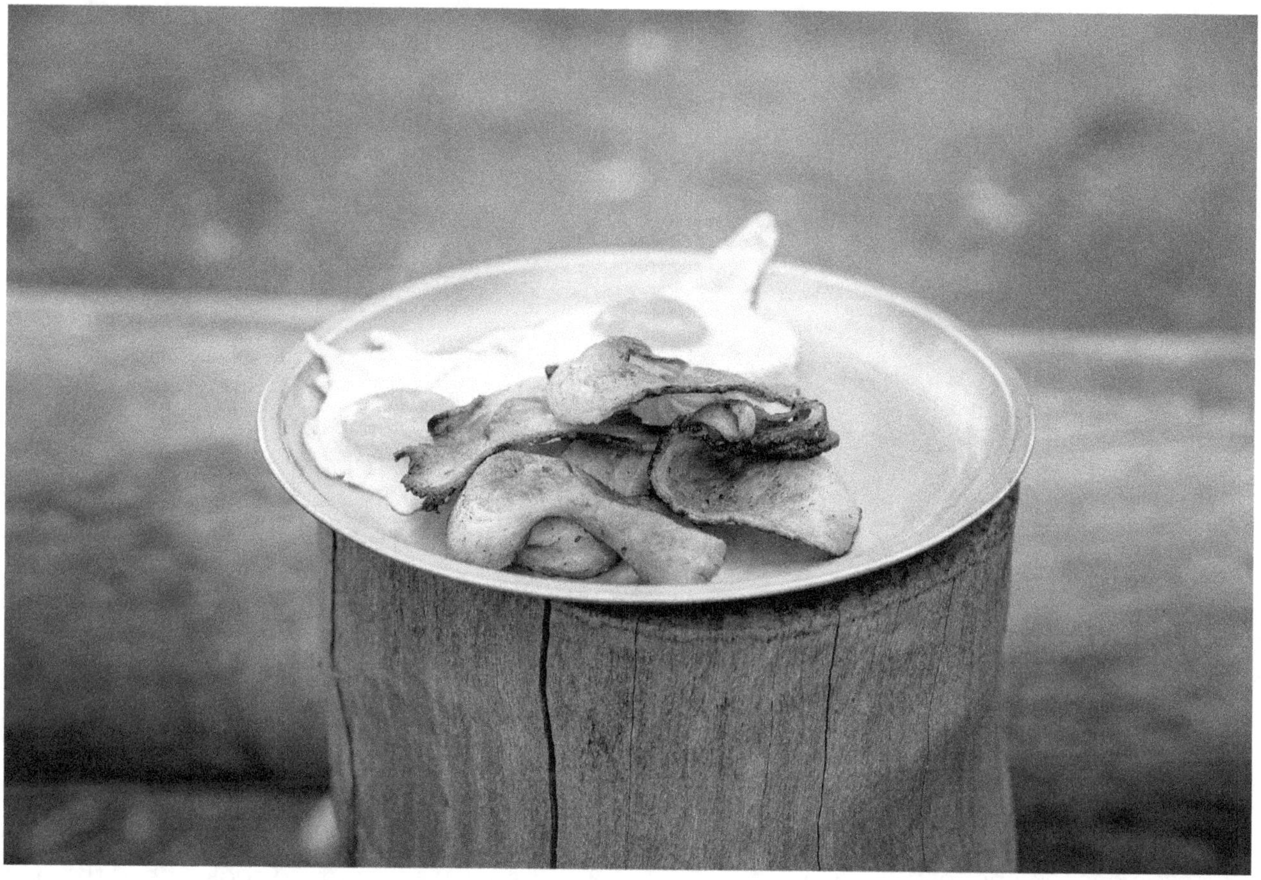

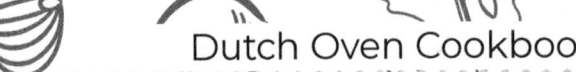
Dutch Oven Cookbook

1. CAMPFIRE BREAKFAST

PREPARATION: 20 MIN **COOKING:** 10 MIN **SERVINGS:** 5

INGREDIENTS

- 4 large eggs and ½ cup milk
- 1 lb. refrigerated hash browns, thawed
- 1 cup chopped ham
- 2 cups shredded cheddar
- ½ tablespoon butter, for greasing the foil

Nutrition: *Calories 442, Fat 22 g, Carbs 35g, Protein 24g*

DIRECTIONS

1. Crack the eggs into a resealable plastic bag and add the milk.
2. Season with salt and pepper.
3. Add the hash browns, ham, and cheese to the bag. Carefully manipulate the bag to combine the ingredients.
4. Butter four squares of aluminum foil.
5. Divide the mixture from the plastic bag between the pieces of foil.
6. Fold it snugly, and seal.
7. Place the packets on a grill or near a campfire, and cook for about 10 minutes.
8. Serve when the eggs are set and the cheese is melted.

2. YUMMY COBBLER

PREPARATION: 20 MIN **COOKING:** 10 MIN **SERVINGS:** 5

INGREDIENTS

- 2 ⅓ cups biscuit mix
- ½ cup sweetened almond milk, vanilla flavor
- ½ tablespoon butter, for coating
- 6 fresh peaches, chopped
- 1 cup strawberries, hulled and chopped

Nutrition: *Calories 118, Fat 12.2 g, Carbs 17g, Protein 8.1 g*

DIRECTIONS

1. Before leaving for camping, combine the biscuit mix and milk in a large, sturdy, resealable bag. Seal the bag.
2. When you are ready to cook, knead the bag with your hands until the ingredients are combined.
3. Butter a large cast iron skillet.
4. Pour in the fruits, and top them with the batter.
5. Cover the pan snugly with foil, and let it cook over the campfire for about 45 minutes.
6. Once the biscuit topping is no longer doughy, the cobbler is ready.
7. Cool for a few minutes before serving.

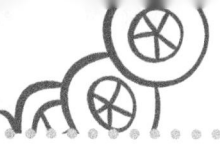 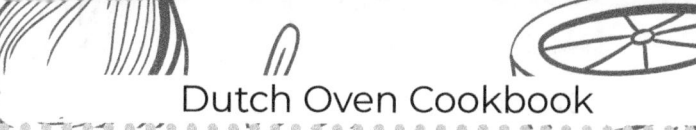

Dutch Oven Cookbook

3. PANCAKES

PREPARATION: 5 MIN   **COOKING:** 20 MIN   **SERVINGS:** 6

INGREDIENTS

- 2 cups pancake mix, plain
- Water, for mixing
- 1 cup blueberries, for topping
- 1 cup bananas, for topping
- 1 cup strawberries, for topping
- 1 cup whipping cream, for topping

DIRECTIONS

1. At home, combine the pancake mix with enough water to make the desired consistency.
2. Pour the batter into a clean condiment bottle, and seal.
3. At the campsite, heat a skillet over the fire or grill.
4. Squeeze some batter onto the pan, cook until bubbles appear, and then flip.
5. When the other side is cooked, serve with the fruit and cream toppings.

Nutrition: Calories 317, Fat 10 g, Carbs 63g, Protein 8.4 g

4. DUTCH OVEN SCRAMBLED EGGS AND BISCUITS RECIPE

PREPARATION: 20 MIN   **COOKING:** 10 MIN   **SERVINGS:** 5

INGREDIENTS

- 1 large onion, chopped
- 1 bell pepper, chopped
- 4 eggs
- 1 package prepared biscuit dough
- ¼ cup cheddar cheese, grated

DIRECTIONS

1. Before leaving for camping, in a large bowl, combine the onion, pepper, eggs, Whisk well.
2. Pour the mixture into any clean condiment bottle, and seal.
3. Prepare the fire using charcoal coals or wood, until the coals are hot enough to cook with.
4. Place the cast iron Dutch oven on the hot coals, and shift the coals around the oven. Let it sit for a few minutes to heat.
5. Add the oil to the oven and let it get hot. Tip the pot so the oil coats the bottom.
6. Pour the egg mixture from the bottle into the Dutch oven. Cover, and let it cook for a few minutes.
7. Grease the lid of the oven with a generous amount of oil and spread it evenly.
8. Open the biscuit package and brush both sides of the rolls with vegetable oil.
9. Place the oiled biscuits on top of the greased oven lid.
10. Place the aluminum foil over the top to keep the heat in.
11. Remove the lid once in a while to stir the eggs, and place it back on again.
12. Once everything is cooked, sprinkle cheese on top of the eggs and let it melt.

Nutrition: Calories 256, Fat 16.6g, Carbs 19.2g, Protein 9.5g

5. EGGS BENEDICT CASSEROLE

PREPARATION: 10 MIN   **COOKING:** 25 MIN   **SERVINGS:** 5

INGREDIENTS

- 6 English muffins, cut into small pieces
- 10 oz. turkey bacon, cut into pieces
- 6 large eggs, or 1 cup egg beaters
- 2 cups milk
- Oil spray for greasing

Nutrition: Calories 302, Fat 9.7g, Carbs 30g, Protein 23g

DIRECTIONS

1. Spray the Dutch oven with oil and set it in the coals to heat.
2. Combine the English muffin pieces with the bacon in the Dutch oven.
3. In a mixing bowl, combine the egg beaters, milk, mustard.
4. Pour this batter on top of the muffin and bacon mixture in the pot, and jiggle the pot so it soaks in evenly.
5. Let it cook until the eggs are set.
6. Serve, and enjoy.

6. DUTCH OVEN EGGS BAKED IN AVOCADOS

PREPARATION: 10 MIN   **COOKING:** 40 MIN   **SERVINGS:** 4

INGREDIENTS

- 4 ripe avocados
- 8 eggs
- Red pepper flakes
- 6 tablespoons hot sauce
- 1 cup salsa

Nutrition: Calories 377, Fat 32g, Carbs 16.4g, Protein 10.6g

DIRECTIONS

1. Slice the avocados and remove the seeds. Scoop out enough of the avocado flesh as needed for the egg to fit. Lay the avocados on a flat surface.
2. Crack an egg into each avocado half.
3. Place all the filled avocados into the Dutch oven.
4. Cover the Dutch oven with the lid and place it on the coals for about 15 minutes, rotating every 5 minutes.
5. Serve with hot sauce and salsa.

7. CAMP QUICHE

PREPARATION: 20 MIN   **COOKING:** 10 MIN   **SERVINGS:** 5

INGREDIENTS

- 6 eggs
- 1 cup broccoli, chopped
- 1 cup mushrooms, chopped
- 1 cup tomatoes, diced
- 1 cup cheddar, shredded

Nutrition: Calories 192, Fat 15.3g, Carbs 3.2g, Protein 11.3g

DIRECTIONS

1. Whisk the eggs in a large mixing bowl, and fold in all the other ingredients EXCEPT the cheese.
2. Pour this mixture into a foil-covered pie plate.
3. Place the pie plate in the Dutch oven, cover, and place the oven over the coals or campfire (on a rack).
4. Cook 25 minutes, or until the eggs are set.
5. Just before serving, sprinkle the cheese over the quiche and let it melt.

8. AUSTRALIAN DAMPER

PREPARATION: 20 MIN **COOKING:** 10 MIN **SERVINGS:** 5

INGREDIENTS

- 3 ½ cups self-rising flour
- 1 tablespoon lemon zest
- Salt, to taste
- ¾ cup almond milk, unsweetened
- 2 teaspoons sugar
- ¼ cup butter
- Pinch cinnamon

Nutrition: Calories 424, Fat 16.5g, Carbs 60g, Protein 8.6g

DIRECTIONS

1. At home, combine all the listed ingredients to make a soft dough, and place it in a large plastic container.
2. To bake the bread, take out the dough from the container and knead it on a clean, floured flat surface until smooth. Shape it into a round loaf.
3. Preheat a Dutch oven over the coals.
4. Grease a sheet of aluminum foil with oil, and dust it with flour.
5. Place the loaf on the foil, and carefully place it in the Dutch oven.
6. Cover, and arrange a few coals on top. Let it cook for about 35 minutes, until it sounds hollow when you tap on the bottom. (Note: if the bottom of the loaf seems to be burning, make a trivet with rolls of foil to lift it off the bottom of the pot.)

9. COUNTRY BREAKFAST

PREPARATION: 20 MIN **COOKING:** 45 MIN **SERVINGS:** 5

INGREDIENTS

- 1 lb. pork sausage
- 2 cups frozen hash browns
- 12 eggs
- 2 cups cheddar cheese, shredded
- 1 container prepared biscuit dough

DIRECTIONS

1. Place the Dutch oven over hot coals and cook the sausages in it until the meat is golden brown. Drain most of the fat.
2. Spoon or shake the prepared hash browns over the sausage.
3. Crack about 12 eggs over the hash browns, and sprinkle on the cheddar cheese.
4. Arrange the biscuits over the cheese.
5. Cover the Dutch oven, and place hot coals on the lid.
6. Cook for 45 minutes, or until the eggs are set.

Nutrition: Calories 446, Fat 29.1g, Carbs 19.4g, Protein 25.7g

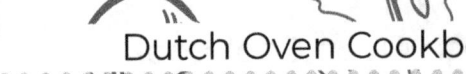

10. BREAKFAST OMELET

PREPARATION: 20 MIN **COOKING:** 30 MIN **SERVINGS:** 5

INGREDIENTS

- 1 tablespoon butter
- 4 slices turkey bacon, chopped
- 8 eggs, beaten
- 1 cup cherry tomatoes, halved
- 1 cup baby spinach, chopped

DIRECTIONS

1. Place a frying pan on a rack over hot coals, and melt the butter in it.
2. Add the turkey bacon and cook for 5 minutes, or until crisp.
3. Pour the eggs into the pan, and add the tomatoes and spinach.
4. When the eggs begin to set, gently left the edge of the omelet and allow the liquid egg to flow under the cooked layer. Repeat until the omelet is set. Do not stir.

Nutrition: Calories 316, Fat, 24g, Carbs 10g, Protein 18.2g

11. CRAB & FENNEL SPAGHETTI

PREPARATION: 10 MIN **COOKING:** 50 MIN **SERVINGS:** 4

INGREDIENTS

- 6 oz. of mixed brown and white crabmeat from sustainable sources
- 1 fresh red chili
- 1 Fennel bulb
- 5 oz. g of dried spaghetti
- 6 oz. of mixed cherry tomatoes

DIRECTIONS

1. Place the Dutch oven on medium-low heat. Trim the fennel, pick any leafy tops and reserve them, then halve the bulb and slice it finely. Put a tbsp. of butter in the oven and cook for 5 minutes with the lid on.
2. Meanwhile, cook the pasta in the Dutch oven of boiling salted water according to the packet instructions, then drain and reserve a mug of the cooking liquid.
3. Slice the chili thinly, stir in the dutch oven and cook uncovered until soft and moist, occasionally stirring.
4. Cut the tomatoes into the oven for 2 minutes, followed by the crab meat and drained pasta 1 minute later. Season with sea salt and black pepper, sprinkle with 1 tablespoon of extra virgin butter, and sprinkle over any reserved fennel tops, if possible, with a splash of the reserved cooking water. Enjoy!

Nutrition: Calories 424, Fat 16.5g, Carbs 60g, Protein 8.6g

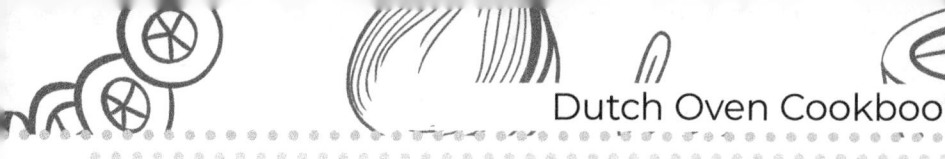

Dutch Oven Cookbook

12. EPIC RIB-EYE STEAK

PREPARATION: 10 MIN   **COOKING:** 30 MIN   **SERVINGS:** 4

INGREDIENTS

- 12 oz. mixed mushrooms
- 4 sprigs of fresh rosemary
- 1 21 oz. jar of quality white beans
- 21 oz. (ideally 5cm thick) piece of rib-eye steak, fat removed
- Four cloves of garlic

Nutrition: Calories 124, Fat 16.5g, Carbs 60g, Protein 8.6g, Sodium 91 mg

DIRECTIONS

1. Place your Dutch oven on medium-high heat.
2. Rub the steak with a pinch of sea salt and black pepper all over, then sear on all sides for a minimum of 10 minutes, so you get a right color on the outside and keep it medium rare in the center, or cook to your liking, occasionally turning with tongs.
3. In the meantime, strip off the sprigs the rosemary leaves, cut and finely slice the garlic and tear any more giant mushrooms.
4. Transfer to a plate when the steak is finished and cover with tin foil.
5. Reduce heat to medium under the Dutch oven and crisp the rosemary for 30 seconds, then add garlic and mushrooms, then you cook for 8 minutes or always toss until golden.
6. Add 1 tbsp. of red wine vinegar and cook for 5 minutes, then season to perfection.
7. Pour over any remaining juices. Slice and serve with a little extra virgin butter at the table, if you like.

13. QUINOA, EVERYDAY DALS, AND AVOCADO

PREPARATION: 10 MIN   **COOKING:** 35 MIN   **SERVINGS:** 4

INGREDIENTS

- 1 Bag Maya Kaimal Everyday Dals of your choosing
- Half cup of quinoa (if you want more quinoa then double the amount of rice and the amount of water)
- 1 avocado
- 1 cup of water

Nutrition: Calories 124, Fat 11.5g, Carbs 60g, Protein 8.6g

DIRECTIONS

1. You're going to use the same pot to heat the Dals and cook the quinoa.
2. Cook the quinoa first. Add the quinoa to the dish, cover with 1 cup of water and a little salt, then bring to a boil. Cover your pot once it has boiled and reduced it to medium-low heat and simmer until the water is absorbed into the quinoa for about 15-20 minutes. Then pass the quinoa to your bowls for cooking.
3. While your oven is still warm, add the Everyday Dals and heat them for about 5 minutes (until they are cooked through), then serve on top of your quinoa.
4. Top with some avocado and enjoy.

14. EASY SAUSAGE CARBONARA

PREPARATION: 5 MIN **COOKING:** 20 MIN **SERVINGS:** 4

INGREDIENTS

- 5 oz. dried tagliatelle.
- Three higher-welfare sausages.
- ½ a bunch of fresh flat-leaf parsley (15g).
- 1 large free-range egg.
- 30 g Parmesan cheese.

Nutrition: Calories 144, Fat 12.5g, Carbs 60g, Protein 8.6g

DIRECTIONS

1. Cook the pasta by following the instructions given to cook the package in the Dutch oven of boiling salted water, then drain and leave a mugful of the cooking liquid.
2. Meanwhile, squeeze out of the skins the sausage meat, then form it quickly into 18 even-sized balls with wet hands.
3. Roll and brush in black pepper, then cook over medium heat in a non-stick frying pan with 0.5 a tablespoon of butter until golden and fried, tossing occasionally, then turn off the heat.
4. Chop the parsley finely, stalks and everything beat it with the egg and a splash of pasta cooking water, then finely grind and mix in most of the Parmesan.
5. Throw the drained pasta into the sausage tub, pour in the egg mixture, and shake off the heat for 1 minute (the residual heat will gently cook the egg).
6. Rinse with a good splash of the reserved cooking water, season with sea salt and pepper to perfection, and finely brush over the remaining Parmesan.

15. BROWN RICE, EVERYDAY DALS, & AVOCADO

PREPARATION: 10 MIN **COOKING:** 30 MIN **SERVINGS:** 4

INGREDIENTS

- 1 cup of water
- 1 Maya Kaimal bag Everyday Dals of your choice
- ½ cup of brown rice
- 1 avocado
- A pinch of salt.

Nutrition: Calories 13, Fat 10.5g, Carbs 60g, Protein 8.6g

DIRECTIONS

1. You're going to use the same pot to cooking both the brown rice and heating the Dals.
2. First, cook the brown rice. Add your rice to the Dutch oven with 1 cup of water and a bit of salt and then bring to a boil.
3. Once boiling, cover your oven and reduce your heat to medium-low and simmer until the water is absorbed into the rice which will take about 15-25 minutes. Then transfer your brown rice into your eating bowls.
4. While your oven is still warm, add the Everyday Dals and warm them up for 5 minutes or until it's heated through, then serve on top of your rice.
5. Top with some cut up avocado and enjoy.
6. Great for: high protein camp meals, quick car camping meals, could make this in a backpacking stove or even make this while backpacking.

16. DUTCH CAMPING FARMERS' BREAKFAST

PREPARATION: 10 MIN **COOKING:** 40 MIN **SERVINGS:** 4

INGREDIENTS

- 6 medium potatoes
- 8 slices bacon
- 1 medium onion, diced
- 6 eggs

DIRECTIONS

1. Cook potatoes in boiling water containing salt until they are finished with their skins.
2. Hot, peel, or put on, cube or slice of skins.
3. Cut bacon into small slices and then fry to desired crispness at medium heat. Drain on the towel of paper.
4. Fry the onions until they are clear enough, add the onions and fry until the crust is shaped. Go back to the bacon.
5. Crack the eggs into the potatoes and then scramble them all around. To taste, add salt and pepper. Pay attention to the salt, as the bacon is salty, together with the parsley.
6. Great as a side dish, brunch, of course, or with a green salad as a main meal for 2.
7. Cooking time is after the cooling of the potatoes.

Nutrition: Calories 428, Fat 13.2g, Carbs 77g, Protein 8.1g

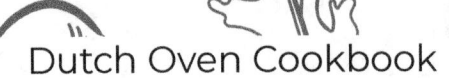

POULTRY

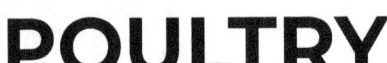

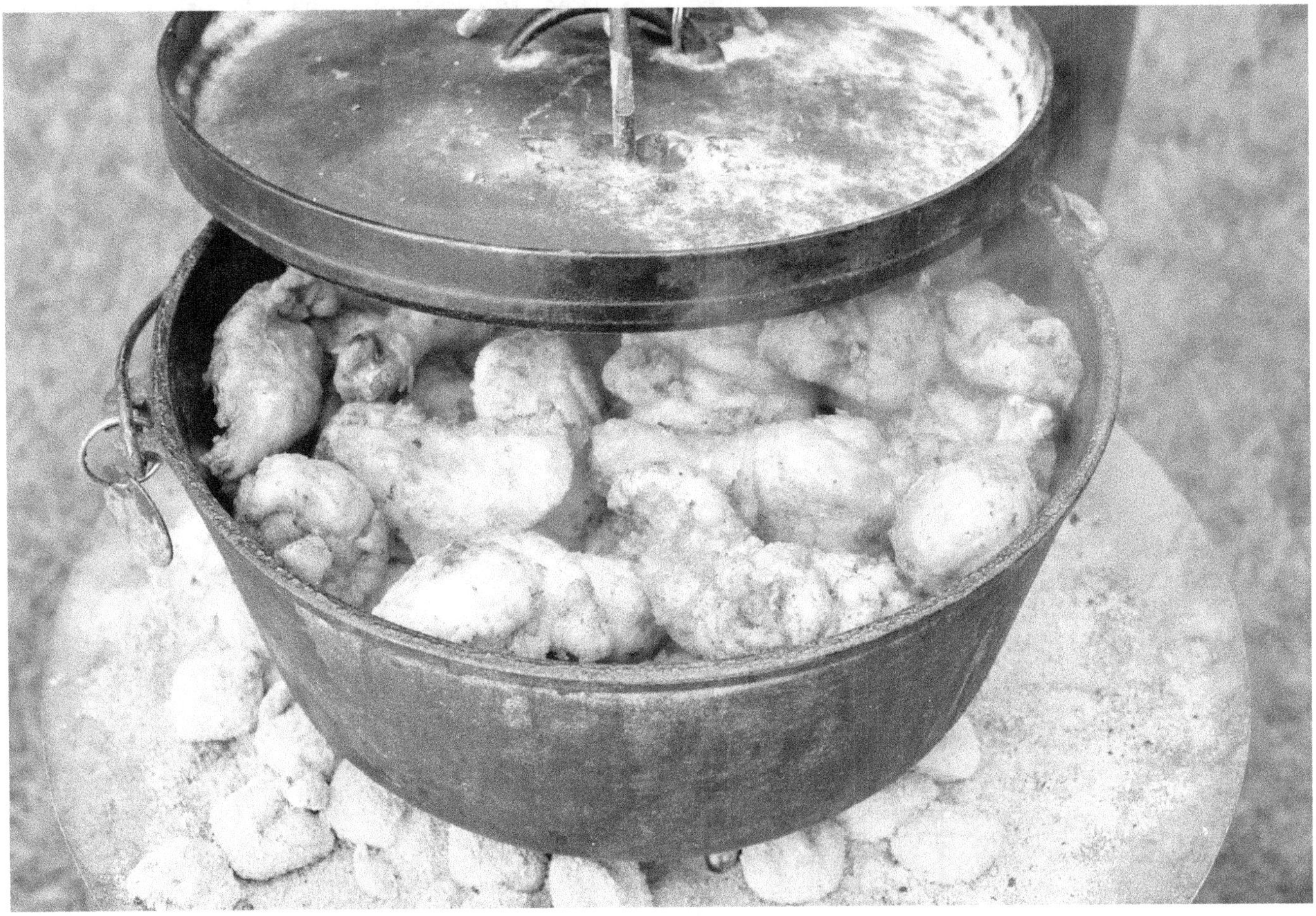

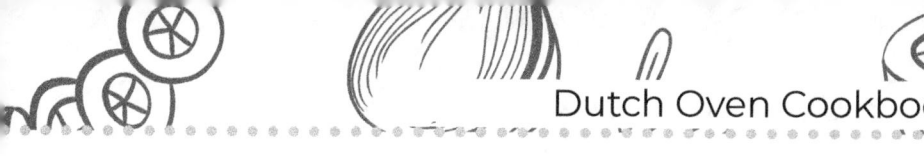

17. CLASSIC CHICKEN "STIR FRY"

PREPARATION: 20 MIN   **COOKING:** 10 MIN   **SERVINGS:** 5

INGREDIENTS

- 4 cups cooked chicken, chopped
- 2 cups rice, cooked
- 1 green bell pepper, sliced
- 1 cup broccoli florets, chopped
- Cooking spray

Nutrition: Calories 514, Fat 5.1g, Carbs 66g, Protein 46g

DIRECTIONS

1. In a large bowl, combine the chicken, rice, green pepper, broccoli. Mix well.
2. Create five double-layer rectangles of foil, and coat them with oil or cooking spray.
3. Divide the chicken mixture among the pieces of foil. Fold up the sides and create packets. Seal well.
4. Place the packets over warm coals for about 15 minutes.

18. BALSAMIC VINEGAR CHICKEN

PREPARATION: 30 MIN   **COOKING:** 10 MIN   **SERVINGS:** 5

INGREDIENTS

- 4 boneless, skinless chicken breast halves
- ¾ cup balsamic vinegar
- ¼ teaspoon soy sauce
- ½ cup pesto
- ½ cup honey mustard sauce

Nutrition: Calories 432, Fat 15g, Carbs 3.4g, Protein 45g

DIRECTIONS

1. Place the chicken, vinegar, soy sauce, salt, and pepper in a Ziploc bag. Let it sit for a few minutes.
2. Heat the grill over medium, and cook the chicken until it is browned on both sides and cooked through.
3. Serve with pesto and honey mustard sauce.

19. CHICKEN OVER THE COALS

PREPARATION: 20 MIN   **COOKING:** 10 MIN   **SERVINGS:** 5

INGREDIENTS

- 1 (4-lb.) fryer chicken
- ½ cup lemon juice
- 2 tablespoons vegetable oil
- 2 teaspoons thyme
- 1 teaspoon rosemary

Nutrition: Calories 548, Fat 17.2g, Carbs 10.2g, Protein 82g

DIRECTIONS

1. Preheat the grill over a hotbed of coals.
2. Cut the chicken into four servings.
3. Remove any skin.
4. Combine the lemon juice, oil, thyme, and rosemary in a bowl, and brush it over the chicken. Season with salt and pepper.
5. Grill the chicken, cavity-side down, and turn after a few minutes.
6. Baste the chicken with the sauce repeatedly while cooking.
7. Once the chicken is golden brown and cooked through, remove it from the heat.

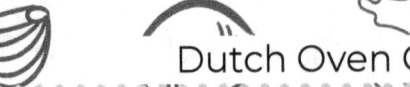
Dutch Oven Cookbook

20. CHICKEN KEBABS

PREPARATION: 50 MIN   **COOKING:** 10 MIN   **SERVINGS:** 5

INGREDIENTS

- 2 lbs. boneless, skinless chicken breasts
- 6 oz. mushrooms, trimmed
- 2 unpeeled oranges, cut into 12 wedges
- ⅓ cup vegetable oil
- 1–2 teaspoons curry powder

Nutrition: Calories 23, Fat 13.5g, Carbs 7.7g, Protein 45g

DIRECTIONS

1. Slice the chicken into long pieces. Thread the pieces on wooden skewers, alternating with mushroom and orange pieces.
2. Once finished, place the skewers in a shallow plastic dish.
3. Pour this mixture over the skewers, making sure they are well coated. Allow them to marinate for 30 minutes.
4. Grill the kebabs over medium coals, turning after 5 minutes.
5. When they are golden brown and cooked through, they are ready to serve.

21. CHICKEN AND POTATOES

PREPARATION: 15 MIN   **COOKING:** 35 MIN   **SERVINGS:** 5

INGREDIENTS

- 5 large chicken breasts
- 5 small potatoes, cut in ½-inch slices
- 1 red onion, chopped
- 1 cup prepared barbecue sauce
- 1 teaspoon sesame seeds

Nutrition: Calories 181 Fat 11, Carbs 47g, Protein 24.6g

DIRECTIONS

1. Shift the coals around the oven.
2. Add the chicken, potatoes, onions, and barbecue sauce, and stir.
3. Cover the oven with the lid and place 12 hot coals on the top. Let it cook for 35 minutes.
4. Once done, serve with a sprinkle of sesame seeds on top.

22. CREAMY SANTA FE CHICKEN

PREPARATION: 5 MIN   **COOKING:** 30 MIN   **SERVINGS:** 4

INGREDIENTS

- 1 lb. chicken tenders
- 1 tablespoon butter
- 2 cup fresh corn kernels
- 2 cups salsa verde (fresh or jarred)
- 1 cup sour cream

Nutrition: Calories 228, Fat 13.2g, Carbs 12g, Protein 38g

DIRECTIONS

1. Preheat oven to 350°F.
2. Add the butter to a skillet and heat over medium.
3. Add the chicken tenders and brown 1-2 minutes per side. Add the corn kernels and cook an additional 2 minutes.
4. Transfer the chicken and corn to a 9"x9" baking dish.
5. Pour the salsa verde over the chicken and bake for approximately 30 minutes. Remove from oven and stir in the sour cream.
6. Serve immediately over rice or in tortilla shells, if desired.

23. MEDITERRANEAN CHICKEN

PREPARATION: 5 MIN   **COOKING:** 30 MIN   **SERVINGS:** 4

INGREDIENTS

- 4 boneless, skinless chicken breasts
- 1 tablespoon butter
- 2 cups cherry tomatoes, quartered
- 1 cup fresh mint leaves, torn
- 1 lemon, juiced and zested

DIRECTIONS

1. Season the chicken breasts with salt and pepper.
2. Heat the butter in sauté pan over medium-high heat. Cook until browned on each side, approximately 5-7 minutes per side, depending upon thickness.
3. Add the tomatoes, mint leaves, lemon juice, and one teaspoon of the lemon zest. Reduce heat to medium and cook, stirring gently, until tomatoes begin to soften. Some of their natural juices are released, approximately 5 minutes.
4. Remove from heat and season with additional salt and pepper, if desired.

Nutrition: Calories 228, Fat 13.2g, Carbs 12g, Protein 38.1g

24. ROSEMARY CHICKEN BAKE

PREPARATION: 5 MIN   **COOKING:** 40 MIN   **SERVINGS:** 4

INGREDIENTS

- 4 bone-in chicken breasts, skin removed
- 1 tablespoon butter
- 2 cups chicken stock
- 1 lemon, sliced
- 2 fresh rosemary sprigs

DIRECTIONS

1. Preheat oven to 375°F
2. Add the butter to a skillet and heat over medium high heat.
3. Add the chicken to the skillet and cook until slightly browned, approximately 3-4 minutes per side.
4. Remove the chicken from the skillet and place in a baking dish. Add ¼ cup of the chicken stock and one rosemary sprig to the chicken. Place in the oven and bake for 25-30 minutes, or until juices run clear.
5. Meanwhile, add the remaining chicken stock, rosemary, and lemon slices to the pan that the chicken was browned in. Turn heat to medium-high and bring to a gentle boil while stirring constantly. Boil for one minute before reducing heat to low. Simmer for ten minutes. Remove rosemary sprig and keep sauce warm over gentle heat.
6. Remove chicken from the oven and transfer to serving plates. Spoon sauce, including lemon slices over each piece of chicken.
7. Serve immediately.

Nutrition: Calories 328, Fat 13.2g, Carbs 3.1g, Protein 18.1g

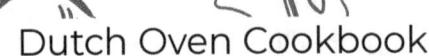
Dutch Oven Cookbook

25. CHICKEN WITH CORNBREAD STUFFING

PREPARATION: 5 MIN   **COOKING:** 4 H   **SERVINGS:** 4

INGREDIENTS

- 4 boneless skinless chicken breasts
- 3 cups dried cornbread crumbs (prepackaged or fresh)
- 2 cups chicken stock
- ½ cup celery, finely diced
- 1 teaspoon dried sage

DIRECTIONS

1. Season the chicken with salt and pepper, then place in a layer among the bottom of the pot.
2. In a bowl, combine the cornbread crumbs, celery, and sage. Add additional salt and pepper, if desired.
3. Add the cornbread mixture over the top of the chicken.
4. Pour the chicken stock over the cornbread mixture, stirring if necessary to make sure corn bread is saturated.
5. Cover the pot and heat on high for 4-6 hours, or until chicken juices run clear.

Nutrition: Calories 388, Fat 13.2g, Carbs 47g, Protein 41g

26. LEEK AND DIJON CHICKEN

PREPARATION: 15 MIN   **COOKING:** 30 MIN   **SERVINGS:** 4

INGREDIENTS

- 4 boneless skinless chicken breasts
- 1 tablespoon butter
- 1 cup leeks, sliced
- 1 tablespoon Dijon mustard
- 1 tablespoon water

DIRECTIONS

1. Preheat oven to 200°F.
2. Add the butter to a large skillet and heat over medium heat. Add the chicken and brown evenly on all sides, approximately 7 minutes per side, depending upon thickness, until juices run clear.
3. Remove chicken from pan and place on an oven safe dish. Place in the oven to keep warm.
4. Add the leeks to the skillet that the chicken was cooked in and sauté over medium heat, stirring and scraping up any chicken residue that remained in the pan. Cook until soft and translucent, approximately 3-5 minutes.
5. In a small bowl, combine the Dijon mustard, and water. Mix well before adding to the pan with the leeks. Warm gently.
6. Remove chicken from the oven and place on serving plates. Top with warm leek and Dijon sauce before serving.

Nutrition: Calories 278, Fat 10.2g, Carbs 7g, Protein 48g

27. ASIAN BBQ CHICKEN

PREPARATION: 15 MIN **COOKING:** 15 MIN **SERVINGS:** 4

INGREDIENTS

- 1 lb. boneless chicken breast, cut into tenders
- 2 tablespoons soy sauce
- 2 tablespoons honey
- 1 teaspoon sesame oil
- 1 tablespoon garlic chili paste

DIRECTIONS

1. Begin by preparing and preheating the grill (either indoor or outdoor grill).
2. In a small bowl, combine the soy sauce, honey, sesame oil, and chili paste. Mix until well blended.
3. Take chicken tenders and gently slide them lengthwise onto metal or bamboo skewers.
4. Baste each skewer with the BBQ sauce.
5. Place skewers on a grill and cook for approximately 10-15 minutes, turning once, until chicken juices run clear. Remove from heat and serve immediately.

Nutrition: Calories 358, Fat 9.3g, Carbs 9g, Protein 48g

28. CHICKEN PICCATA

PREPARATION: 5 MIN **COOKING:** 25 MIN **SERVINGS:** 4

INGREDIENTS

- 4 boneless, skinless chicken breasts
- ¼ cup butter
- 1 cup dry white wine
- ¼ cup lemon juice
- 3 tablespoons capers
- 1 teaspoon salt
- 1 teaspoon pepper

DIRECTIONS

1. Preheat oven to 200°F.
2. Begin by gently pounding the chicken breasts until they are approximately ¼-inch thick. Season with salt and pepper.
3. Over medium-high heat, add the butter to a large sauté pan. Add the chicken and brown evenly on both sides, approximately 5-7 minutes per side, until juices run clear.
4. Transfer chicken, leaving remaining butter in the sauté pan, an oven-safe dish, and place in the oven to keep warm.
5. Add the dry white wine to the pan and reduce over medium heat for approximately 10 minutes, scraping the bottom of the pan occasionally to loosen any bits remaining from the chicken.
6. Add the lemon juice and capers. Cook for another 2 minutes.
7. Remove the chicken from the oven and place back in the pan. Heat through, spooning the sauce over the chicken for 1-2 minutes.
8. Transfer to serving plates and serve immediately.

Nutrition: Calories 328, Fat 23.2g, Carbs 16g, Protein 48g

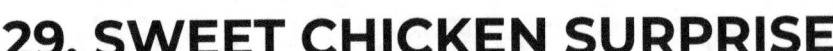

Dutch Oven Cookbook

29. SWEET CHICKEN SURPRISE

PREPARATION: 10 MIN **COOKING:** 30 MIN **SERVINGS:** 3

INGREDIENTS

- 2 x 7 oz. g free-range chicken legs
- 1 bulb of garlic
- 9 oz. mixed-color seedless grapes
- 100 ml red vermouth
- Four sprigs of fresh tarragon

DIRECTIONS

1. Preheat the oven to 360°F.
2. Put Dutch oven on high heat. Rub the chicken all over with a ½ t a tbsp. of butter, season with black pepper and salt with the skin side down in the Dutch oven.
3. Fry for few minutes until golden, then lightly squash the unpeeled garlic cloves with the heel of your hand and add. Pick in the grapes.
4. Turn the chicken skin side up, pour in the vermouth, transfer to the oven to roast for 40 minutes, or until the chicken is golden and tender. The sauce is sticky and reduced.
5. Add a little water to the pan and give it a gentle shimmy to pick up all the sticky bits. Pick over the tarragon, and dish up.

30. THAI RED CHICKEN SOUP

PREPARATION: 10 MIN **COOKING:** 120 MIN **SERVINGS:** 3

INGREDIENTS

- 1 butternut squash (42 oz.)
- 3.5 oz. Thai red curry paste
- 3.5 lb whole free-range chicken
- 1 bunch of fresh coriander (30g)
- 1 x 400 milliliter tin of light coconut milk

DIRECTIONS

1. Sit in a big, deep pan with the chicken.
2. Carefully halve the length of the squash, then cut the seeds into 3 cm chunks.
3. Slice the stalks of coriander, add the squash, curry paste, and coconut milk to the Dutch oven, and then pour 1 liter of water. Cover and cook for 1 hour and 20 minutes at medium heat.
4. Use tongs to remove a platter from the chicken. Sprinkle some fat on the chicken from the soup sheet, then sprinkle with half the leaves of coriander.
5. Serve at the table with 2 forks to split the meat. Crush some of the squash using a potato masher, giving a thicker texture to your soup.
6. Taste, season to perfection with black pepper and salt, then divide between six bowls and sprinkle with the remaining coriander.
7. Add chicken and Shred, as you dig in.

Nutrition: Calories 118, Fat 7.2g, Carbs 17g, Protein 8.1g

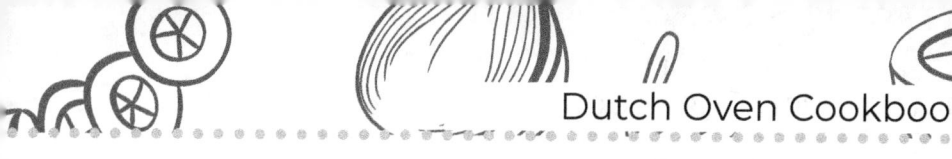

31. CHICKEN IN A POT

PREPARATION: 10 MIN **COOKING:** 5 H **SERVINGS:** 3

INGREDIENTS

- 3-4 lb. whole frying chicken
- 1 tsp. poultry seasoning
- 1/4 tsp. basil

DIRECTIONS

1. Wash chicken and pat dry. Sprinkle cavity with poultry seasoning. Put in the Dutch oven and sprinkle with basil. Cover and bake for about 5 hours or until tender.

32. EASY CHICKEN DINNER

PREPARATION: 10 MIN **COOKING:** 30 MIN **SERVINGS:** 3

INGREDIENTS

- 2 Chickens
- Carrots
- Seasonings
- Flour
- Potatoes

DIRECTIONS

1. Cut vegetables and potatoes for eating into small pieces. Split eight pieces of the chicken. Chicken of the back. In a plastic bag, mix the flour and seasonings. Put 2 pieces of chicken in the bag at a time and shake.
2. Once coated, remove the chicken from the bag and repeat until all the chicken has been eaten. Place and shake the potatoes in the bag. Cut from the bag the vegetables.
3. In the Dutch oven, add around 1/2 inches of oil and put on the coals. Add chicken and brown on all sides when the oil is hot. Drain excess oil from the pot and remove the chicken from the dish. Return the chicken to the bowl.
4. Apply around 1/4 inch warm water. Place over chicken potatoes and vegetables. Cover the pot and place it on the coals.
5. Set on top of the oven, ten coals. Cook until chicken is tender for 1 hour. Check regularly to ensure that a small amount of moisture is always present in the Dutch oven.

Nutrition: Calories 238, Fat 13.2g, Carbs 27g, Protein 38.1g

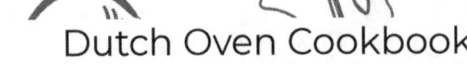

33. EASY CHICKEN CASSEROLE

PREPARATION: 10 MIN   **COOKING:** 30 MIN   **SERVINGS:** 3

INGREDIENTS

- 1 Whole chicken cooked, chopped
- 2 cans Cream of Chicken Soup or 1 can Golden Mushroom soup
- 1 cup Mayonnaise
- 1 box "Stove Top" stuffing, chicken flavor
- Cheddar cheese

DIRECTIONS

1. Combine soup and mayonnaise in a massive bowl of choice. Then season pkg from stuffing mix and ¾ stuffing crumb.
2. Add chicken and mix well. Place in the Dutch oven, and then you top with remaining crumbs. Bake at 350°F for 30 min until bubbly and crumbs are brown. Variation change 1 can Golden Mushroom soup with Cream of Chicken soup. Add shredded cheddar cheese in soup mixture depending on your choice. You can sprinkle on it.

Nutrition: Calories 318, Fat 23.2g, Carbs 13g, Protein 8.1g

---

34. SCRAMBLED EGG OMELETTE

PREPARATION: 10 MIN   **COOKING:** 30 MIN   **SERVINGS:** 3

INGREDIENTS

- 12 oz. ripe mixed-color tomatoes
- ½-1 fresh red chili
- ½ a bunch of fresh basil (1/2 oz.)
- Four large free-range eggs
- ½ x 5 Oz. ball of mozzarella

DIRECTIONS

1. Slice the tomatoes thinly, place on a sharing tray, then dress with a little extra virgin butter, red vinegar, sea salt, and black pepper.
2. Put most of the basil leaves into a pestle and mortar, pound into a paste with a pinch of salt, then muddle extra virgin butter in 1 tablespoon to make basil oil.
3. Slice the chili finely. Cut the mozzarella perfectly.
4. Put the Dutch oven with half a tablespoon of butter on medium heat. Beat and pour in the eggs, stir periodically with a rubber spatula, gently pushing the eggs around the Dutch oven.
5. Stop the stir and scatter the mozzarella at the center when they are gently scrambled but still loose, then drizzle over the basil oil.
6. Let the bottom of the rest of the egg for 1 minute, then use the spatula to flip it back to the center, then fold the top half back over as well. Turn it to the tomato platter upside down, right side up.
7. Slice down the center to reveal in the middle the oozy scrambled eggs. Scatter (as much as you dare!) over the chili and the remaining basil leaves, and tuck in.

Nutrition: Calories 338, Fat 15.2g, Carbs 7g, Protein 10.1g

VEGETARIAN AND SIDE DISH RECIPES

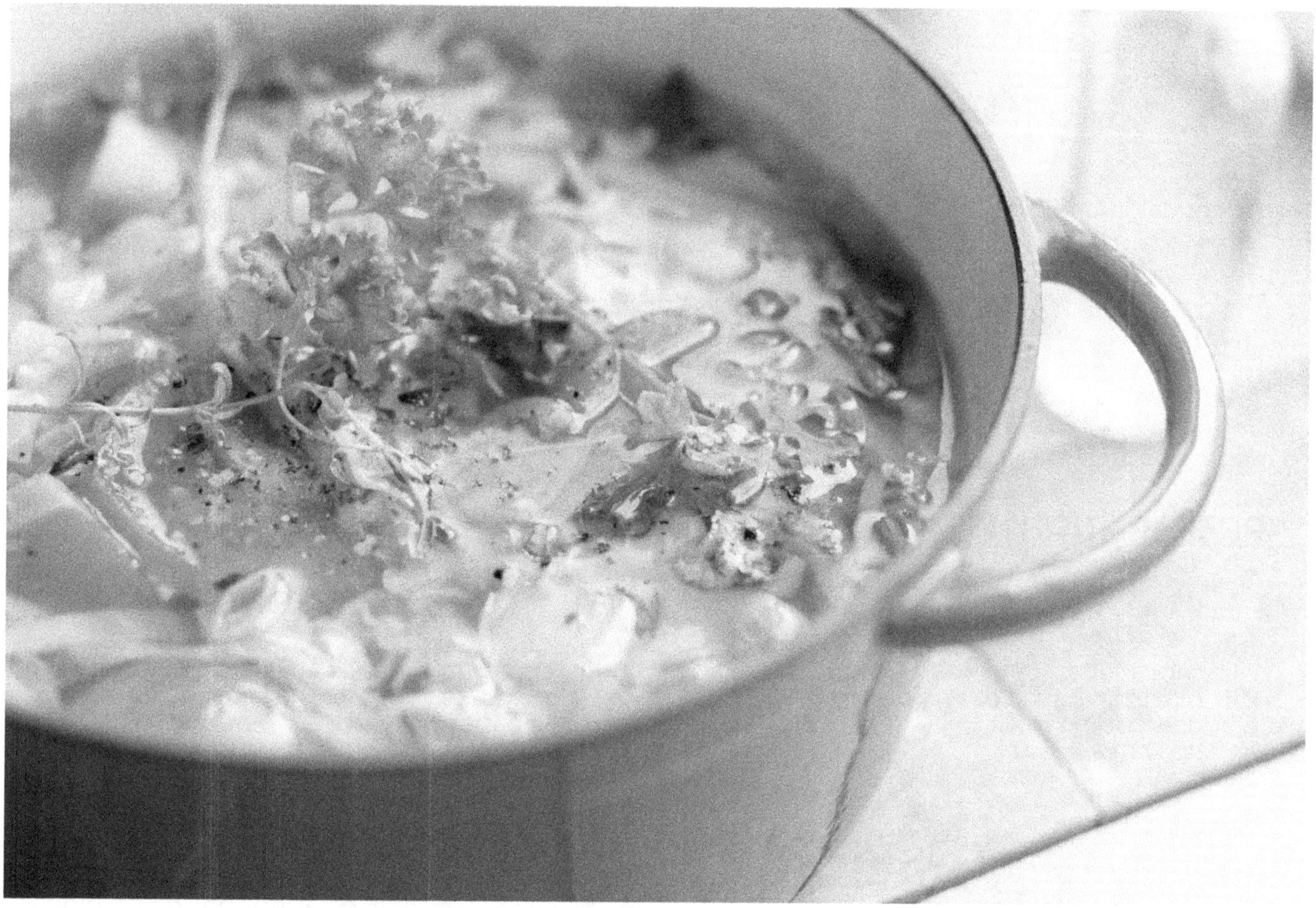

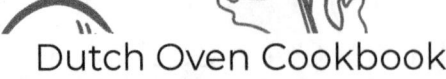
Dutch Oven Cookbook

35. DUTCH POTATO AND EGG SCRAMBLE

PREPARATION: 10 MIN   **COOKING:** 25 MIN   **SERVINGS:** 4

INGREDIENTS

- 2 Diced Medium Potatoes
- 8 Eggs stirred
- 1 Chopped Onion
- 2 Tablespoons Butter

DIRECTIONS

1. This is a healthy breakfast is an easy meal for campers, and a great way to start the day. It cooks up in 1 pot and serves about four.
2. First, add 1 Tbs of Butter into your Dutch oven and put it over your fire. Melt it and spread it around.
3. Second, add Potatoes, Onions, and Peppers. Chuck the potatoes and for the Onion and Peppers to be chopped, but it's your choice.
4. Cook these until the Potatoes are tender, and the Onions is sweet and cooked. Cook for about 20 minutes, but it depends on the supplied heat.
5. Third, add the second tbsp. of butter and, once it's melted, add the Eggs. The Eggs fills all the spaces in between the Potatoes, Peppers, and Onions. So cover the oven and let it cook until the eggs are beautiful and ready for about 4 minutes to ensure even cooking time.

Nutrition: Calories 328, Fat 15.2g, Carbs 10g, Protein 4.1g

36. DUTCH OVEN MOUNTAIN MAN

PREPARATION: 10 MIN   **COOKING:** 25 MIN   **SERVINGS:** 4

INGREDIENTS

- 2 lb. sausage
- 2 lb. of frozen hash brown potatoes
- 8 eggs, beaten
- 1/4 cup water
- 2 cups grated cheese

DIRECTIONS

1. Fry and crumble the sausage in a Dutch oven. Once cooked, remove the sausage and drain it using paper towels.
2. Brown potatoes using the drippings from the sausage in the pan and spread on the bottom of the oven evenly.
3. Place the previously cooked sausage atop the potatoes and pour in the eggs over the sausage layer. Top with cheese.
4. There should be 16 coals on the lid and eight under the oven. Cook the eggs for 20-25 minutes.

Nutrition: Calories 438, Fat 18.2g, Carbs 56g, Protein 11.2g

37. DUTCH OVER POTATOES WITH CHEESE

PREPARATION: 10 MIN **COOKING:** 30 MIN **SERVINGS:** 4

INGREDIENTS

- 8 Potatoes
- 1 package of cooked and crumbled bacon
- 2 cups shredded cheese
- 1 cup of onions

DIRECTIONS

1. Slice your potatoes thin pieces and the onion into rings. Chop the bacon as well as add it to a preheated Dutch oven. Cook the bacon and scoop it out after it cooks, leaving the grease at the bottom of the Dutch oven.
2. Layer the potatoes, onions, bacon, and cheese, respectively and repeated these layers. Cover the Dutch oven and leave to cook at 375°F for around 45 minutes until the potatoes turn soft.

Nutrition: Calories 235, Fat 16.4g, Carbs 12g, Protein 6.9g

38. DUTCH OVEN RAVIOLI

PREPARATION: 10 MIN **COOKING:** 20 MIN **SERVINGS:** 4

INGREDIENTS

- 1 25 oz. bag frozen sausage ravioli, thawed
- 1 sizeable 45 oz. jar spaghetti sauce
- ¼ cup fresh Parmesan cheese (can use grated)
- 1 cup shredded Mozzarella cheese
- ½ cup water

DIRECTIONS

1. Spray the Dutch oven or cover it with tin foil sprayed with cooking spray. At the bottom of a 1-2" Dutch oven, put a thin layer of spaghetti sauce then place a single layer of the ravioli on top.
2. On the ravioli, pour half of the remaining spaghetti sauce and sprinkle with the Parmesan cheese. Add another layer of ravioli on top of the sauce and pour in the rest of the spaghetti sauce.
3. Use the mozzarella cheese to top the sauce and add a little Parmesan cheese. To add moisture, pour the water around the edges of the pan — Cook in the Dutch oven for 45 minutes at 350°F. The cheese should start to brown, and the sauce should be bubbling.

Nutrition: Calories 338, Fat 14g, Carbs 57g, Protein 7g

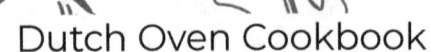
Dutch Oven Cookbook

39. GRILLED SWEET POTATO FRIES

PREPARATION: 10 MIN **COOKING:** 20 MIN **SERVINGS:** 3

INGREDIENTS

- 2 Medium Sweet Potatoes
- 2 Tablespoons Butter or Vegetable Oil
- 1 Clove of Garlic, Chopped
- 1 Teaspoon Chili Powder
- 1 A packet of Ranch Dry Mix

Nutrition: Calories 138, Fat 9.4g, Carbs 28g, Protein 7g

DIRECTIONS

1. Wash the Sweet Potatoes and dry them. Then cut them in lengthwise strips, about 1/3 an inch wide on each side, so they look like fries.
2. The important thing is that they must be uniform so they can cook up at the same time. If you wanted to produce a crispier fries, and you have the time, soak the chips in water for about 30 minutes and then let drain for an hour before continuing. If otherwise, then that's fine too, they'll still be delicious.
3. Mix all the recipe ingredients in a bowl. We want all the beautiful spices and dry mix to be uniformly covered. Place the Dutch oven on a grate over an open fire or on the middle rack of a grill.
4. We're going to cook the potatoes and make them soft and crispy on the outside. You want about ten minutes per side, depending on your heat flipping once.

40. BLISTERED SHISHITO PEPPERS

PREPARATION: 10 MIN **COOKING:** 20 MIN **SERVINGS:** 3

INGREDIENTS

- ½ lb. Shishito Peppers
- 2 garlic cloves, sliced into chips
- 2 tablespoons oil
- 1 large shallot, thinly sliced

Nutrition: Calories 146, Fat 5g, Carbs 3g, Protein 0g

DIRECTIONS

1. Oil and garlic chips to a cold Dutch oven, and turn the heat on to medium. This will allow garlic to infuse the oil with flavor.
2. Observe the garlic chips, and remove from the oil with a slotted spoon just when they begin to brown. It happens quickly, and they are easy to burn. Set aside.
3. Turn the heat up to medium-high, and add the peppers to the hot garlic oil. They will crackle and blister. Turn them occasionally until they are dried and blistered all over. You may have to remove smaller ones before larger ones.
4. Sprinkle the top with garlic chips, and either serve warm or pack in a jar for enjoying later.

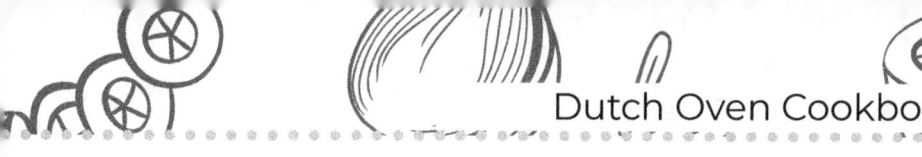

41. BUBBLE AND SQUEAK

PREPARATION: 10 MIN **COOKING:** 35 MIN **SERVINGS:** 3

INGREDIENTS

- 1 small head of cabbage or 1/2 large head, chopped
- Five medium potatoes, sliced in bite-size wheels
- 1 or 2 Polish or Kielbasa type sausages (all kinds I tried were great, even bulk sausage!)
- 1 cup of water
- Butter

DIRECTIONS

1. Get 1 pot (Dutch oven), layer chopped cabbage, potatoes, sausage, and then repeat until all ingredients are used.
2. Add water and butter, cover, and simmer until cabbage and potatoes and sausages are cooked. Probably about 15 or 20 minutes.

Nutrition: Calories 128, Fat 11.4, Carbs 21g, Protein 11g

42. SIZZLING SEARED SCALLOPS

PREPARATION: 10 MIN **COOKING:** 20 MIN **SERVINGS:** 3

INGREDIENTS

- 7 oz. frozen peas
- 14 oz. potatoes
- ½ a bunch of fresh mint (15g)
- 6-8 raw king scallops (coral attached, trimmed, from sustainable sources)
- 2 oz. firm higher-welfare black pudding

DIRECTIONS

1. Wash the potatoes, chop into 3 cm chunks and cook for 1-2 minutes or until tender, adding the peas for the rest 3 minutes in the Dutch oven of boiling salted water.
2. Meanwhile, most of the mint leaves are picked and finely chopped and put aside.
3. Place 1 tablespoon of butter and leaves the remaining mint to crisp for 1 minute, then scoop the leaves onto a plate and leave the oil behind.
4. Season the scallops on each side for 2 minutes or until golden with sea salt and black pepper. Crumble it in the black pudding (so it chips next to each other).
5. Drain the potatoes and peas, return to the oven, properly mash with the chopped mint and 1 tablespoon of extra virgin butter, taste, and season.
6. Layer with the scallops and black pudding and sprinkle lightly with extra virgin butter.

Nutrition: Calories 421, Fat 16g, Carbs 27g, Protein 9g

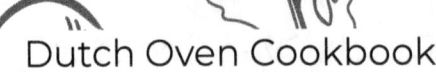

43. PAN TOASTED COUSCOUS

PREPARATION: 5 MIN **COOKING:** 30 MIN **SERVINGS:** 4

INGREDIENTS

- 2 cups chicken stock
- 1¼ cup couscous
- 1 tablespoon butter
- ¼ cup shallots, diced
- 1 lemon, juiced and zested

DIRECTIONS

1. Add the chicken stock to a saucepan and bring to a boil over medium high heat.
2. Add the couscous and stir. Remove from heat, cover and let sit 5-7 minutes, or until all liquid has been absorbed.
3. In a large sauté pan, heat the butter over medium heat. Add the shallots and cook for 2 minutes. Add 1 tablespoon of lemon juice and 2 teaspoons of lemon zest. Stir and cook for 1 minute.
4. Add the couscous into the sauté pan and increase the heat to high. Cook, stirring often for 10 minutes. Reduce the heat to medium-low and cook, occasionally stirring for 20 minutes.
5. Remove from heat and serve immediately.

Nutrition: Calories 148, Fat 7g, Carbs 21g, Protein 3g

44. FRESH CUCUMBER SALAD

PREPARATION: 5 MIN **COOKING:** 0 MIN **SERVINGS:** 4

INGREDIENTS

- 3 cups cucumber, cubed
- 1½ cups watermelon, cut into small cubes
- ½ cup red onion, sliced
- ½ cup fresh cilantro, chopped
- 2 teaspoons fresh lime juice

DIRECTIONS

1. In a large bowl, combine the cucumber, watermelon, and red onion.
2. Season with cilantro, lime juice, salt and pepper. Mix well.
3. Place in the refrigerator and chill for at least 2 hours.
4. Stir well before serving.

Nutrition: Calories 214, Fat 3g, Carbs 11g, Protein 1g

45. SWEET ROASTED ROOT VEGETABLES

PREPARATION: 5 MIN **COOKING:** 30 MIN **SERVINGS:** 4

INGREDIENTS

- ¼ cup butter, melted
- 2 cups carrots, chopped
- 1 cup sweet potato, diced
- 1 cup rutabaga, diced
- ¼ cup wildflower honey

DIRECTIONS

1. Preheat oven to 400°F.
2. In a bowl, combine the carrots, sweet potato, and rutabaga.
3. Drizzle the vegetables with melted butter and honey. Season with salt and pepper. Toss well to coat.
4. Spread the vegetables out on a baking sheet. Place in the oven and bake for 30-35 minutes, or until vegetables are tender and caramelized.

Nutrition: Calories 264, Fat 11, Carbs 24g, Protein 5.4g

46. FENNEL GRATIN

PREPARATION: 10 MIN **COOKING:** 60 MIN **SERVINGS:** 4

INGREDIENTS

- 3 cups fennel, sliced
- ¾ cup vegetable stock
- ¼ cup butter
- 1 cup fine bread crumbs
- 1 cup fresh grated parmesan cheese
- 1 teaspoon salt
- 1 teaspoon pepper

DIRECTIONS

1. Preheat oven to 375°F.
2. Place the fennel slices in a lightly oiled 8"x8" baking dish. Cover with chicken stock and 2 tablespoons of butter cubed. Season with salt and pepper.
3. Cover and place in the oven. Bake for 35 minutes.
4. Meanwhile, in a small saucepan, melt the remaining butter. Add in the breadcrumbs, parmesan cheese, and additional salt and pepper, if desired.
5. Remove gratin from the oven and top with bread crumb mixture.
6. Recover the dish and place back in the oven. Bake for an additional 30-35 minutes, or until fennel is tender.
7. Let rest 5 minutes before serving.

Nutrition: Calories 326, Fat 12g, Carbs 29g, Protein 9g

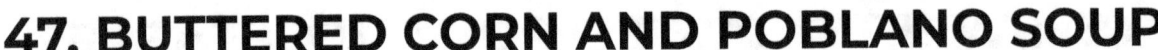
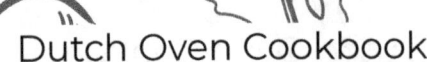

47. BUTTERED CORN AND POBLANO SOUP

PREPARATION: 5 MIN **COOKING:** 30 MIN **SERVINGS:** 4

INGREDIENTS

- 1 tablespoon butter
- 4 cups fresh corn kernels
- 2½ cups milk
- 1 cup Monterey Jack cheese, shredded

DIRECTIONS

1. In a Dutch oven, melt the butter over medium heat. Add the corn kernels and cook while stirring for approximately 3-4 minutes, or until corn is slightly toasted.
2. Add the milk and bring the mixture to a boil over medium-high heat for two minutes. Season with salt and pepper.
3. Transfer one half of the soup to a blender and pulse until creamy and thick. Return to the Dutch oven and mix well.
4. Gently reheat soup over low heat.
5. Serve immediately topped with Monterey jack cheese.

Nutrition: Calories 291, Fat 19.8g, Carbs 10g, Protein 7g

48. PITA PIZZA BLANCO

PREPARATION: 10 MIN **COOKING:** 15 MIN **SERVINGS:** 4

INGREDIENTS

- 4 pieces of pita bread
- ¾ cup crème fraiche
- 3 cloves garlic, crushed and minced
- ½ cup fresh oregano, chopped
- 1½ cup fresh mozzarella cheese, sliced

DIRECTIONS

1. Preheat oven to 420°F.
2. Spread out the pita bread pieces on one or two baking sheets.
3. In a bowl, combine the crème fraiche, garlic, and oregano. Blend well.
4. Spread the mixture evenly on each of the pita breads. Top with several slices of fresh mozzarella cheese.
5. Place in the oven and bake for 15 minutes, or until cheese is golden and bubbly.
6. Serve warm.

Nutrition: Calories 413, Fat 26g, Carbs 41g, Protein 7.4g

49. ANCIENT GRAIN STUFFED PEPPERS

PREPARATION: 5 MIN **COOKING:** 35 MIN **SERVINGS:** 4

INGREDIENTS

- 4 large red bell peppers, tops removed and seeds scooped out
- 3 cups ancient grain blend, cooked
- 1 tablespoon butter
- 2 cups white mushrooms, sliced
- ½ cup fresh parsley, chopped

DIRECTIONS

1. Preheat oven to 350°F.
2. In a large bowl combine the ancient grains, butter, mushrooms, and parsley. Season with salt and pepper as desired.
3. Stuff each pepper liberally with the mixture and replace the tops of the peppers.
4. Transfer the peppers to a baking dish and add 1 tablespoon of water to the dish's bottom.
5. Place in the oven and bake for 35-40 minutes, or until peppers are tender.
6. Serve immediately.

Nutrition: Calories 318, Fat 15g, Carbs 39g, Protein 11g

50. PARMESAN RISOTTO

PREPARATION: 10MIN **COOKING:** 35 MIN **SERVINGS:** 4

INGREDIENTS

- 1 large shallot, finely chopped
- 2 quarts low-sodium vegetable or chicken broth, at room temperature
- 2 cups Arborio, carnaroli, or vialone nano rice
- ½ cup dry white wine
- 1 cup Parmesan cheese, finely grated

DIRECTIONS

1. Add the butter to the Dutch oven and melt it over medium-high heat.
2. Mix in the rice until mixed well with the butter. Stir-cook for about 2 minutes until lightly toasted and aromatic.
3. Mix in the wine and simmer for 3 minutes until the wine is almost completely reduced and nearly dry.
4. Pour in the broth ½ cup at a time, stirring with each addition.
5. Cook for 20–30 minutes until the mixture is thickened and the rice is al dente.
6. Add some more butter and cheese, if desired.
7. Serve warm.

Nutrition: Calories 465, Fat 11g, Carbs 66g, Protein 20g

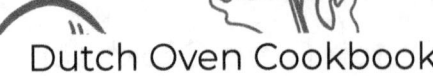

51. ALL-TIME FAVORITE MAC AND CHEESE

PREPARATION: 5 MIN **COOKING:** 35 MIN **SERVINGS:** 4

INGREDIENTS

- 3 cups of water
- 3½ cups whole milk
- 1 lb. elbow macaroni
- 4 oz. Velveeta, cubed
- 2 cups sharp cheddar, shredded

DIRECTIONS

1. Add the water, milk, and pasta to the Dutch oven. Stir and heat over medium-high heat.
2. Reduce heat to medium-low and simmer, stirring occasionally, for 12–15 minutes until the mixture is thickened and the pasta is tender.
3. Mix in the Velveeta and cheese and simmer over low heat until melted.
4. Serve warm.

Nutrition: Calories 344, Fat 14g, Carbs 39g, Protein 16g

52. CREAMY MUSHROOM PASTA

PREPARATION: 5 MIN **COOKING:** 15 MIN **SERVINGS:** 4

INGREDIENTS

- 2 tablespoons butter
- ¾ lb. mixed mushrooms (shiitake, cremini, oyster, etc.), sliced
- 3 cloves garlic, minced
- 1-quart chicken, mushroom, or vegetable broth
- Grated Parmesan cheese

DIRECTIONS

1. Add the oil to the Dutch oven and heat it over medium-high heat.
2. Add the mushrooms and stir cook for about 4 minutes until lightly browned.
3. Add the garlic, cream, pasta, and broth and stir-cook for a few seconds.
4. Bring to a boil, and then reduce heat to low and simmer for about 12 minutes, stirring occasionally, until the pasta is cooked well and the mixture is thickened.
5. Serve warm with thyme and grated Parmesan on top.

Nutrition: Calories 607, Fat 26g, Carbs 71g, Protein 20g

Dutch Oven Cookbook

53. MASCARPONE PUMPKIN PASTA

PREPARATION: 5 MIN **COOKING:** 15 MIN **SERVINGS:** 4

INGREDIENTS

- 1 cup canned pumpkin puree
- 1-quart vegetable broth
- 1 cup of water
- ¾ lb. dry penne pasta
- 2 teaspoons fresh rosemary leaves, finely chopped

DIRECTIONS

1. Add the pumpkin puree, broth, water, and pasta to the Dutch oven and bring to a boil over medium-high heat.
2. Reduce heat to low and simmer for 10–12 minutes until most of the liquid evaporates, stirring occasionally.
3. Mix in the mascarpone, rosemary
4. Stir-cook for about 2 minutes until the pasta is cooked to your satisfaction.
5. Serve warm with grated Parmesan on top.

Nutrition: Calories 245, Fat 4g, c 43g, Protein 8g, Sodium 63 mg

54. CLASSIC CHEESY SPAGHETTI

PREPARATION: 10 MIN **COOKING:** 12 MIN **SERVINGS:** 4

INGREDIENTS

- ½ cup of water
- 1-quart chicken broth
- ¾ lb. dry spaghetti
- 1 Parmesan cheese rind (optional)
- ¾ cup Pecorino-Romano cheese, grated

DIRECTIONS

1. Add the water, broth, and pasta and Parmesan rind to the Dutch oven and bring to a boil over medium-high heat.
2. Simmer for 8–9 minutes until most of the liquid evaporates, stirring occasionally.
3. Mix in the Pecorino-Romano
4. Stir-cook for 2 minutes until the pasta is cooked to your satisfaction.
5. Remove the Parmesan rind.
6. Serve warm.

Nutrition: Calories 497, Fat 10.5g, Carbs 73.5g, Protein 25g

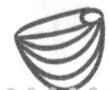 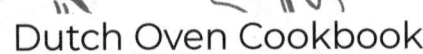
Dutch Oven Cookbook

55. BRAISED LEEKS

PREPARATION: 15 MIN **COOKING:** 50 MIN **SERVINGS:** 4

INGREDIENTS

- 6 medium leeks (white portion and light green parts only), halved lengthwise
- ¼ cup butter
- 1 teaspoon dry rosemary (or 2 teaspoons fresh rosemary)
- 2 teaspoons sugar
- ½ cup dry white wine

DIRECTIONS

1. Preheat the oven 350°F.
2. Clean the leeks under cold running water to remove any remaining dirt.
3. Add the butter in the Dutch oven, and let melt over medium-low heat. Add the leeks and brown them on the cut side down for 2-3 minutes over medium heat.
4. Turn the leeks over, add the remaining ingredients. Stir to combine. Cover and place in the oven. Bake for 35-45 minutes checking midway to turn over the leeks back cut side down. Add a bit of water if needed to prevent the leeks from sticking to the bottom.
5. Remove from the oven once the leeks are tender. If there is lots of cooking juice, you can reduce it on the stove, uncovered, over medium-high heat until most of the liquid has evaporated.

Nutrition: Calories 153, Fat 5g, Carbs 18g, Protein 3g

56. FRENCH ONION PASTA

PREPARATION: 10 MIN **COOKING:** 35 MIN **SERVINGS:** 4

INGREDIENTS

- 3 tablespoons butter
- 1½ lbs. yellow onions, sliced paper-thin
- ⅔ Cup water
- 1-quart low-sodium vegetable or beef broth
- ¾ lb. dry orecchiette pasta
- ⅓ cup ruby port
- 2 oz. (about ¾ cup) Gruyere cheese, finely shredded
- Salt and pepper to taste

DIRECTIONS

1. Add the oil to the Dutch oven and heat it over medium-high heat.
2. Add the onion slices and stir-cook for 15–20 minutes until caramelized and dark.
3. Add the water, broth, pasta, and ruby port; stir and cook for 12 minutes until the liquid is evaporated.
4. Mix in the Gruyere. Season to taste with salt and pepper.
5. Serve warm.

Nutrition: Calories 520, Fat 12g, Carbs 84g, Protein 17.5g

57. SEASONED FRENCH FRIES

PREPARATION: 5 MIN **COOKING:** 60 MIN **SERVINGS:** 4

INGREDIENTS

- 3 lbs. russet potatoes, cut into ½-inch sticks
- 3 quarts peanut oil
- 2 teaspoons Old Bay seasoning

DIRECTIONS

1. Add the potato sticks to a bowl and cover with cold water; set aside for 30–60 minutes. Drain and pat dry.
2. Add the peanut oil to the Dutch oven and heat it to 325°F.
3. In 2–3 batches, fry the potato sticks for 7–9 minutes until golden brown.
4. Drain over paper towels.
5. Increase heat to 400°F.
6. Return the cooked potato sticks to the Dutch oven in 2–3 batches and fry for 1–2 minutes until deep golden brown.
7. Drain over paper towels. Serve warm.

Nutrition: Calories 226, Fat 7g, Carbs 39g, Protein 5g

58. BUTTERY CARROTS

PREPARATION: 10 MIN **COOKING:** 10 MIN **SERVINGS:** 4

INGREDIENTS

- 1 cup of water
- 2 lbs. carrots cut into 2-inch pieces
- ⅓ Cup butter
- 2 tablespoons all-purpose flour
- 2 teaspoons chicken bouillon granules

DIRECTIONS

1. Pour 1 inch of water into the Dutch oven.
2. Add the carrots and boil for 6–8 minutes until tender. Drain and set aside.
3. Add the butter and melt it over medium-high heat.
4. Add the onion and stir-cook until softened and translucent.
5. Add the flour and bouillon
6. Bring to a boil and then simmer for about 2 minutes until the mixture is thickened, stirring occasionally.
7. Stir in the carrots. Serve

Nutrition: Calories 129, Fat 8g, Carbs 14g, Protein 2g, Sodium 416 mg

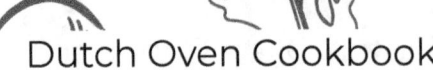
Dutch Oven Cookbook

59. BAKED GARLIC AND MUSHROOM RICE

PREPARATION: 10 MIN   **COOKING:** 40 MIN   **SERVINGS:** 4

INGREDIENTS

- 3 tablespoons butter
- 1 lb. mushrooms, diced
- 3 cloves garlic, minced
- 1½ cups of rice
- ½ cup white wine

DIRECTIONS

1. Warm the butter in the Dutch oven over medium heat.
2. Stir in the diced mushrooms and minced garlic.
3. Cook for about 10 minutes and then stir in the rice.
4. Pour in the white wine and cook for 2 minutes. Pour in the water, bring to a boil, and cover.
5. Bake at 350°F for about 25 minutes.
6. Remove the lid and cook uncovered for 5 minutes until the rice is set and nicely baked.

Nutrition: Calories 406, Fat 11.3g, Carbs 63.3g, Protein 9g

60. QUINOA WITH MIXED VEGETABLES AND ARTICHOKE HEARTS

PREPARATION: 5 MIN   **COOKING:** 40 MIN   **SERVINGS:** 4

INGREDIENTS

- 3 tablespoons butter
- 2 cloves garlic, minced
- 1 (14 oz.) bag of frozen vegetables
- ½ cup artichoke hearts, diced
- 2 cups quinoa, washed and rinsed

DIRECTIONS

1. Warm the butter in the Dutch oven over medium heat.
2. Stir in the minced garlic, frozen veggies, and diced artichoke hearts.
3. Cook for 5 minutes and then stir in the quinoa.
4. Pour in the water and bring to a simmer.
5. Reduce heat to low, cover, and cook for 20 minutes.
6. Remove the lid and mix everything to fluff up the quinoa with the veggies.
7. Serve on plates.

Nutrition: Calories 490, Fat 15.9g, Carbs 72.8g, Protein 15.9g

61. DUTCH OVEN VEGETARIAN LASAGNA

PREPARATION: 5 MIN   **COOKING:** 40 MIN   **SERVINGS:** 4

INGREDIENTS

- 5 tablespoons butter
- 4 cups baby spinach
- ½ lb. lasagna sheets
- 1 (28 oz.) can tomato sauce
- 4 cups grated mozzarella cheese

DIRECTIONS

1. Warm the butter in the Dutch oven over medium heat.
2. Stir in the baby spinach.
3. Cook for 5 minutes until the spinach wilts.
4. Stir in the tomato sauce and cook for 5 minutes.
5. Remove from heat and transfer all but a little of the filling to a bowl.
6. Add a layer of lasagna sheets to the Dutch oven.
7. Add a layer of the filling and sprinkle with mozzarella cheese.
8. Repeat at least two more times or until you run out of lasagna sheets and filling.
9. Sprinkle the top with mozzarella cheese and pepper.
10. Cover and bake at 350°F for about 20 minutes.
11. Remove the lid and cook uncovered for about 15 more minutes until the mozzarella is golden brown.
12. Let cool slightly, then slice and serve.

Nutrition: Calories 490, Fat 24g, Carbs 54.6g, Protein 19.3g

62. CHEESY RAVIOLI PASTA BAKE

PREPARATION: 5 MIN   **COOKING:** 40 MIN   **SERVINGS:** 4

INGREDIENTS

- 3 tablespoons butter
- 1 lb. mushrooms, diced
- 4 (9 oz.) packages spinach ravioli
- 1 (24 oz.) jar marinara sauce
- ½ lb. mozzarella cheese, shredded

DIRECTIONS

1. Warm the butter in the Dutch oven over medium heat. Add the diced mushrooms.
2. Stir in the marinara sauce.
3. Let the flavors marry together and then add the ravioli.
4. Bring to simmer and transfer the Dutch oven to a preheated oven at 350°F.
5. Bake for 25–30 minutes.

Nutrition: Calories 747, Fat 37.4g, Carbs 69.3g, Protein 36.1g

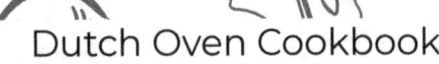

63. VEGETARIAN JAMBALAYA

PREPARATION: 5 MIN **COOKING:** 35 MIN **SERVINGS:** 4

INGREDIENTS

- 2 tablespoons butter
- 1 (14 oz.) bag of frozen vegetables
- 2 (16 oz.) cans red beans, drained and rinsed
- 1 cup long-grain rice
- 1 (28 oz.) can diced tomatoes

DIRECTIONS

1. Warm the butter in the Dutch oven over medium heat.
2. Stir in the frozen veggies and cook for 5–7 minutes.
3. Stir in the rice and cook for 2–3 minutes.
4. Stir in the diced tomatoes and water.
5. Mix and bring to a boil.
6. Reduce heat to low and simmer, covered, for 20 minutes.
7. Stir in the red beans and serve warm.

Nutrition: Calories 1113, Fat 9.9g, Carbs 202.2g, Protein 59.4g

64. STUFFED ZUCCHINI

PREPARATION: 20 MIN **COOKING:** 40 MIN **SERVINGS:** 5

INGREDIENTS

- 2 tablespoons butter
- 2 large onions, chopped
- 1 cup quinoa, rinsed
- 1 cup cannellini beans, drained
- ½ cup almonds, chopped

DIRECTIONS

1. Place a cast iron Dutch oven over the campfire or hot coals.
2. Heat the oil and sauté the onions.
3. Add the quinoa and water.
4. Bring the mixture to a boil, put on the lid, and let it cook for 10 minutes.
5. Transfer this cooked quinoa to a bowl, and add the beans and almonds.
6. Cut the zucchini lengthwise, and scoop out the seeds.
7. Fill the zucchinis with the quinoa stuffing.
8. Wipe out the Dutch oven with paper towel, and spray it with cooking spray.
9. Arrange the zucchinis in the Dutch oven. Cover, and place it over the heat.
10. If you're using charcoal, then put some coals on the lid.
11. Cook it about 25–30 minutes.
12. When the zucchinis are fork tender, serve.

Nutrition: Calories 407, Fat 13.2g, Carbs 58g, Protein 18.5g

SOUP AND STEW

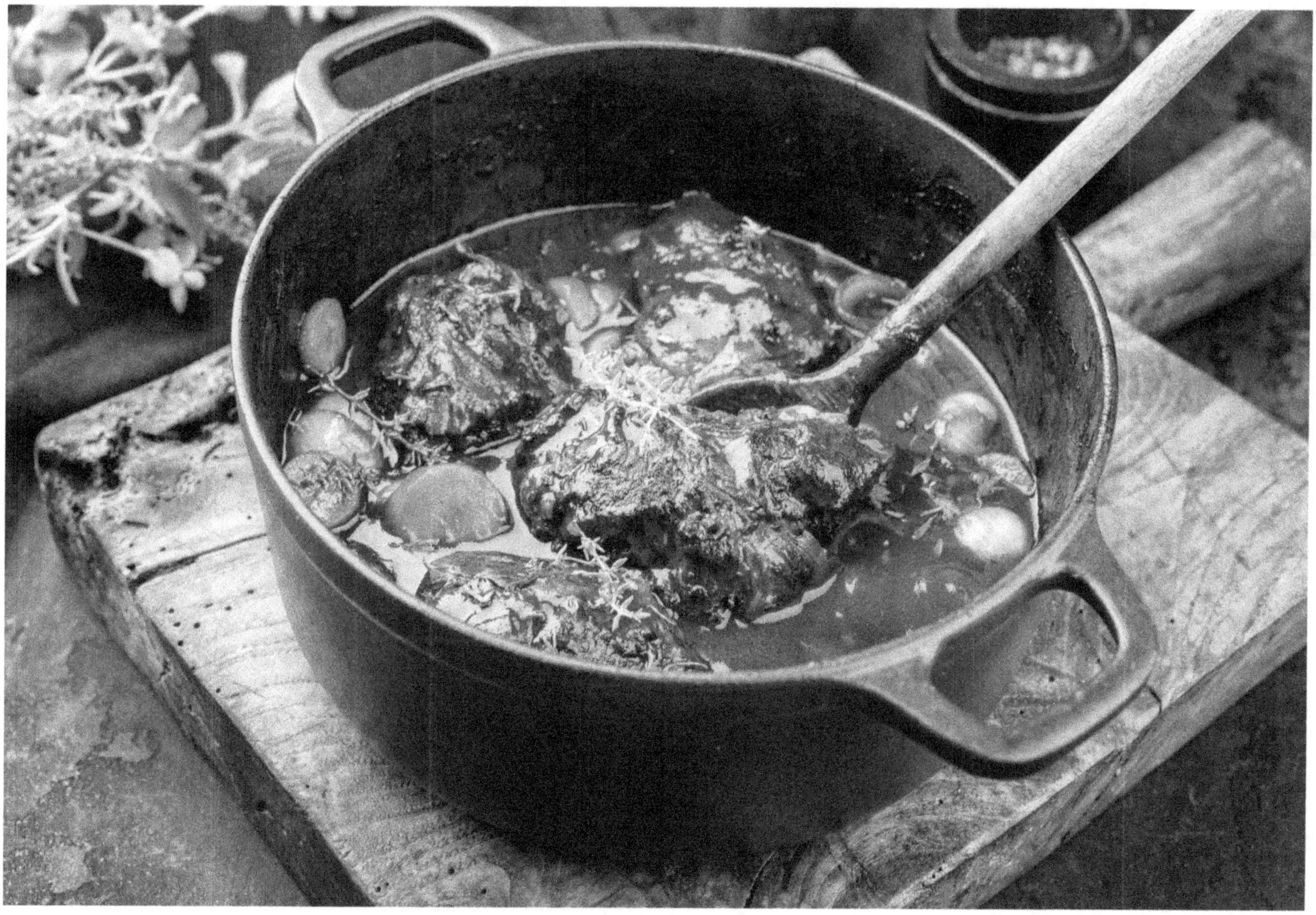

65. VEGETABLE STEW

PREPARATION: 5 MIN   **COOKING:** 40 MIN   **SERVINGS:** 4

INGREDIENTS

- 5 tablespoons butter
- 2 (14 oz.) bags frozen mixed vegetables
- ½ lb. mushrooms halved
- 2 potatoes, peeled and cut into 1-inch cubes
- 1 (14 oz.) can tomato sauce

DIRECTIONS

1. Warm the butter in the Dutch oven over medium heat.
2. Stir in the frozen vegetables, mushrooms, and diced potatoes and cook for 5–7 minutes.
3. Stir in the tomato sauce and water.
4. Bring to a boil and cook for 30 minutes.
5. Remove half of the diced potatoes to a plate and mash them with a fork.
6. Return them to the Dutch oven and stir to thicken the stew.
7. Serve

Nutrition: Calories 400, Fat 18.3g, Carbs 52.5g, Protein 10.9g

---

66. STUFFED BELL PEPPERS

PREPARATION: 20 MIN   **COOKING:** 30 MIN   **SERVINGS:** 5

INGREDIENTS

- 6 large bell peppers, tops off, seeds removed
- 2 tablespoons vegetable oil
- 1 lb. ground beef
- 2 cups white rice, (cooked at home)
- ½ cups tomato sauce

DIRECTIONS

1. Place the Dutch oven in the coals to heat.
2. Add the vegetable oil, beef, and cook until brown.
3. Add the tomato sauce and precooked rice, and mix well.
4. Spoon the filling into the cored bell peppers. Wipe out the oven with paper towel.
5. Arrange the stuffed bell peppers in the Dutch oven, and cover. Place some coals on the lid.
6. Bake for 20 to 30 minutes, until the peppers are tender.
7. Serve and enjoy.

Nutrition: Calories 480, Fat 10g, Carbs 66g, Protein 30.5g

67. SAUSAGE, PEPPER & POTATO PACKETS

PREPARATION: 20 MIN   **COOKING:** 25 MIN   **SERVINGS:** 5

INGREDIENTS

- 3 red potatoes, cut in chunks
- 4 cooked dinner sausages, sliced
- 2 onions, sliced
- 2 tablespoons butter
- ½ teaspoon paprika

DIRECTIONS

1. Mix all the ingredients together in a large bowl.
2. Cut a long piece of heavy-duty foil into a 12x20 inch rectangle, and coat it with cooking spray.
3. Place the mixture in the center of the foil and enclose it to form a package.
4. Cook the packet a few inches above the coals, on a grill rack, turning it twice.
5. After 25 minutes, check that the potatoes are cooked through. Serve!

Nutrition: Calories 434, Fat 22.5g, Carbs 30.3g, Protein 24g

68. CHICKEN MUSHROOM SOUP

PREPARATION: 10 MIN   **COOKING:** 25 MIN   **SERVINGS:** 5

INGREDIENTS

- 2 celery ribs, chopped
- 1-quart chicken broth
- ⅓ cup all-purpose flour
- 2 cups cooked chicken, cubed
- 1 (8¾ oz.) package precooked chicken-flavored rice

DIRECTIONS

1. Add the oil to the Dutch oven and heat it over medium-high heat.
2. Add the vegetables and stir-cook until the carrots become soft, crisp, and tender.
3. Add the broth and flour to a mixing bowl. Mix well.
4. Pour the broth into the Dutch oven and bring to a boil, stirring occasionally.
5. Stir-cook for 5–6 minutes until thickened.
6. Add the other ingredients and cook over medium-low heat until cooked to satisfaction.
7. Serve warm.

Nutrition: Calories 224, Fat 7g, Carbs 23g, Protein 15g

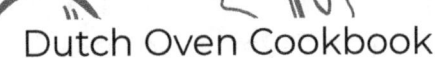

69. CREME POTATO CHICKEN SOUP

PREPARATION: 10 MIN **COOKING:** 10 MIN **SERVINGS:** 5

INGREDIENTS

- 3½ cups water
- 4 cups shredded cooked chicken breast
- 2 (10¾ oz.) cans condensed cream of chicken soup, undiluted
- 1 lb. frozen mixed vegetables, thawed
- 1 (14½ oz.) can potatoes, drained and diced

DIRECTIONS

1. Add the water, chicken breast, chicken soup, vegetables, and potatoes to the Dutch oven. Bring to a boil.
2. Reduce heat to low, cover, and simmer for 8–10 minutes until the veggies are tender, stirring occasionally.
3. Mix in the cheese.
4. Serve warm with minced chives on top.

Nutrition: Calories 429, Fat 22g, Carbs 23g, Protein 33g

70. BEEF AND CABBAGE SOUP

PREPARATION: 20 MIN **COOKING:** 120 MIN **SERVINGS:** 5

INGREDIENTS

- 1 lb. beef stew meat, cut into ¾-inch pieces
- 2 tablespoons butter
- 6 cups beef stock, divided
- 1 medium-sized green cabbage, shredded
- 1 ½ teaspoon Italian seasoning

DIRECTIONS

1. Pat the beef dry with paper towels
2. Add butter to a large Dutch oven and sear the meat over medium heat on all sides until well browned. Do not overcrowd the oven, work in batches if needed. Place the browned beef on a plate.
3. Add about half of the beef stock and bring to a boil. Stir and scrape the brown bits. Return the beef to the Dutch oven.
4. Add the cabbage, tomatoes, onion, remaining beef stock, water, garlic, Italian seasoning.
5. Bring to a boil over medium-high heat.
6. Decrease the heat to medium-low and let cook for 2 hours until the beef is tender and cabbage soft, taking care of stirring a few times.
7. Taste and adjust seasoning with salt and pepper.

Nutrition: Calories 176, Fat 3g, Carbs 15g, Protein 13g

71. QUINOA CHICKPEA CORN SOUP

PREPARATION: 20 MIN **COOKING:** 25 MIN **SERVINGS:** 10

INGREDIENTS

- 1 tablespoon butter
- 1–2 jalapeño peppers, seeded and chopped (optional)
- 2 quarts vegetable broth
- 1 cup fresh or frozen corn
- 2 (15 oz.) cans unsalted chickpeas or garbanzo beans, rinsed and drained

DIRECTIONS

1. Add the oil to the Dutch oven and heat it over medium-high heat.
2. Mix in the quinoa and broth.
3. Bring to a boil.
4. Reduce heat to low and simmer for about 10 minutes until the quinoa is tender, stirring occasionally.
5. Serve warm with chopped cilantro on top if desired.

Nutrition: Calories 289, Fat 5g, Carbs 48g, Protein 13g

72. SWEET POTATO SOUP

PREPARATION: 10 MIN **COOKING:** 125 MIN **SERVINGS:** 5

INGREDIENTS

- 4 sweet potatoes, peeled and diced
- 2 (14 oz.) can of light coconut milk
- 2 cup vegetable broth
- 4 cloves garlic, minced
- 2 teaspoon dried basil

DIRECTIONS

1. Place all the ingredients in the Dutch oven and stir.
2. Cover and cook for 1 hour 30 minutes, or until the sweet potatoes are tender.
3. Puree with an immersion blender until the soup is smooth.

Nutrition: Calories 127, Fat 5g, Carbs 20g, Protein 1g

73. PORK AND BEAN SOUP

PREPARATION: 20 MIN **COOKING:** 55 MIN **SERVINGS:** 5

INGREDIENTS

- 1-quart water
- 3 cups pork roast, cooked and cubed
- 1 (15 oz.) can navy beans, rinsed and drained
- 2 medium potatoes, peeled and chopped
- Minced fresh basil (optional)

DIRECTIONS

1. Add the water, pork roast, beans, potatoes, and remaining ingredients to the Dutch oven.
2. Bring to a boil.
3. Reduce heat to low, cover, and simmer, stirring occasionally, for 40–45 minutes until the roast is cooked to perfection and veggies are tender and crisp.
4. Serve warm with minced basil on top.

Nutrition: Calories 206, Fat 5g, Carbs 23g, Protein 18g

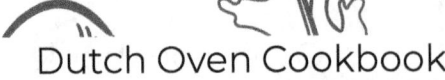
Dutch Oven Cookbook

74. TOMATO CREAM SOUP WITH BASIL

PREPARATION: 20 MIN　　**COOKING:** 125 MIN　　**SERVINGS:** 5

INGREDIENTS

- 3 large carrots, peeled
- 2 celery stalks
- 2 medium onions
- 1-quart chicken broth, low sodium
- ½ cup fresh basil leaves, roughly chopped, more for serving

DIRECTIONS

1. Dice the carrots, celery, and onions.
2. Bring to a boil, cover, reduce heat to low, and cook for 2 hours or until the vegetables are soft and tender.
3. Use an immersion blender to puree.
4. Serve garnished with more basil leaves, if desired.

Nutrition: Calories 180, Fat 5g, Carbs 31g, Protein 5g

75. CHICKEN BEAN BARLEY SOUP

PREPARATION: 20 MIN　　**COOKING:** 20 MIN　　**SERVINGS:** 5

INGREDIENTS

- 2 strips thick-cut bacon
- 1 cup dried barley, soaked overnight, rinsed, and drained
- 1 ½ cups dried navy beans, soaked overnight, rinsed and drained
- 6 cups low-sodium chicken broth
- 1 small rotisserie chicken, skin removed, and meat shredded

DIRECTIONS

1. Brown the bacon in the Dutch oven over medium heat. When crisp, drain and transfer to a plate lined with paper towels. Set aside.
2. Drain off the drippings, leaving about 1 tablespoon.
3. Place the barley and beans in the Dutch oven.
4. Pour in the broth and water, and stir.
5. Bring to a boil over medium-high heat. Cover, reduce heat to medium-low, and cook 60-75 minutes until beans and barley are tender. Check a few times and add more water if needed.
6. Add the chicken continue cooking for another 20 minutes.
7. Crumble the reserved bacon. Serve warm with some of the bacon on top.

Nutrition: Calories 149, Fat 3g, Carbs 15g, Protein 16g

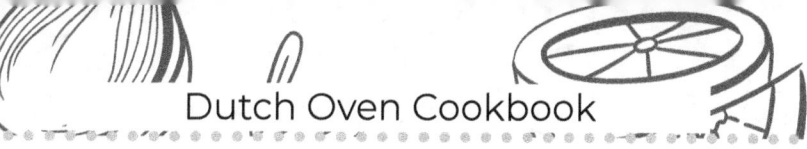

76. COLLARD GREEN WHITE BEAN SOUP WITH SAUSAGES

PREPARATION: 20 MIN **COOKING:** 125 MIN **SERVINGS:** 5

INGREDIENTS

- 1 lb. dried white beans, soaked overnight, rinsed, and drained
- ½ lb. Cajun Andouille sausages, sliced
- 4 sprigs fresh thyme
- 8 cups chicken broth, low-sodium
- 8 cups collard greens, leaves only, cut into 1-inch pieces

DIRECTIONS

1. Place the beans in a Dutch oven and cover with water.
2. Bring to a boil over high heat. Reduce heat to medium-low, cover, and cook for 45-50 hours or until the beans are tender. Remove from heat and drain the water.
3. Add the sausages, onion, celery, thyme, and chicken broth. Bring a boil over high heat, reduce heat to low, cover and cook for 30 minutes over medium-low heat.
4. Remove the thyme stems and drop in the collard greens. Cover and cook 15-20 minutes longer or until the greens are tender.
5. Serve

Nutrition: Calories 393, Fat 8g, Carbs 51g, Protein 30g

77. BACON AND POTATO SOUP

PREPARATION: 20 MIN **COOKING:** 75 MIN **SERVINGS:** 5

INGREDIENTS

- 8 strips bacon
- 2 teaspoons bacon drippings or butter
- 3 lbs. potatoes, peeled, cut into ¼-inch slices
- 2 (14 ½ oz.) cans chicken broth, Fat-free, lower-sodium
- ¾ cup cheddar cheese, shredded, more for serving

DIRECTIONS

1. Fry the bacon strips in the Dutch oven until crispy over medium heat, about 4-5 minutes. Remove the bacon and place on a plate lined with paper towels.
2. Keep about 2 tablespoons of the bacon drippings (or oil) in the Dutch oven. Add butter if necessary. Warm the drippings over medium heat, and stir-fry the onions until tender. Remove from heat.
3. Place the potato slices in the Dutch oven. Stir in the water, broth, salt, and pepper and stir.
4. Cover and cook for 40-45 minutes over medium-low heat or until the potatoes are tender.
5. Mash potatoes with a potato masher or blender stick. Stir in milk and cheese. Stir to combine.
6. Let simmer over low heat for about 20-25 minutes or until heated through and smooth.
7. Serve with sour cream, sprinkled with bacon, chives, more cheese, if desired.

Nutrition: Calories 259, Fat 6g, Carbs 38g, Protein 13g

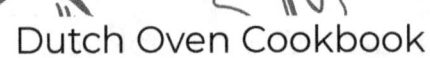
Dutch Oven Cookbook

78. VEGETABLE SOUP

PREPARATION: 20 MIN **COOKING:** 45 MIN **SERVINGS:** 5

INGREDIENTS

- 4 cups chicken or vegetable stock
- 3 medium potatoes
- 2 yellow sweet potato
- 2 celery stalks
- 3 carrots

DIRECTIONS

1. Wash and peel the vegetables, and then cut them into bite-size chunks.
2. Place the vegetables and stock in your Dutch oven, add in about 2 cups of water. The vegetables should be covered with liquid up to an inch.
3. Bring the ingredients to a boil, lower the heat and simmer for 35-40 minutes or until the vegetables are tender and cooked through.
4. Purée using a stick blender and serve hot. You can garnish with sour cream, cream, black pepper if you wish.

Nutrition: Calories 158, Fat 5.2g, Carbs 31g, Protein 2g

79. JERUSALEM ARTICHOKE SOUP

PREPARATION: 10 MIN **COOKING:** 15 MIN **SERVINGS:** 5

INGREDIENTS

- 4 tablespoons cream
- 2 cups milk
- 18 oz. Jerusalem artichokes

DIRECTIONS

1. Peel the Jerusalem artichokes and chop them.
2. In your Dutch oven, add the milk and cream and bring to a boil. Once done, add the Jerusalem artichokes and simmer until soft; this should take about 15 minutes.
3. Remove from heat and use a hand blender to blend until smooth.
4. You can top with chopped chives if you wish.

Nutrition: Calories 279, Fat 15, Carbs 16g, Protein 5

80. BLACK BEAN SOUP

PREPARATION: 10 MIN **COOKING:** 15 MIN **SERVINGS:** 5

INGREDIENTS

- 1 teaspoon chili powder
- 1 teaspoon cumin
- 1 cup vegetable broth
- 16 oz. salsa
- 2 (15 oz.) cans black beans, drained

DIRECTIONS

1. In a large Dutch oven, mix 1 can of beans, chili powder, vegetable broth, salsa and cumin. You can add your favorite spices at this point if you wish. Stir well and bring the ingredients to a boil. Cook for 10 minutes while stirring from time to time.
2. Once ready, use an immersion blender to blend the ingredients.
3. Add the remaining 1 can of beans and cook for 5 more minutes; season with salt.
4. Serve warm. You can serve with cilantro and avocado if you wish.

Nutrition: Calories 158, Fat 13.2g, Carbs 77g, Protein 8.1g, Sodium 896 mg

81. CORN AND BLACK BEAN SOUP

PREPARATION: 3 MIN **COOKING:** 5 MIN **SERVINGS:** 5

INGREDIENTS

- 1 (14.4 oz.) can no-salt added diced tomatoes
- 1 (14.4 oz.) can fat-free refried beans
- 1 (14.4 oz.) can black beans, drained and rinsed
- 1 (14.4 oz.) can corn, drained and rinsed
- 1 (14.4 oz.) can fat-free chicken broth

DIRECTIONS

1. Mix all the ingredients in a Dutch oven and stir well.
2. Simmer and then serve. You can garnish with green onions, sour cream and avocado if you wish.

Nutrition: Calories 283, Fat 11g, Carbs 31g, Protein 12g

82. POTATO SOUP

PREPARATION: 10 MIN **COOKING:** 25 MIN **SERVINGS:** 5

INGREDIENTS

- 1 cup shredded sharp cheddar, plus extra for serving
- 2 tablespoons Cajun seasoning
- 2 lbs. fresh Russett potatoes, cubed or shredded
- 5-6 cups chicken or vegetable broth
- 6 green onions, thinly sliced with white and green parts separated

DIRECTIONS

1. In a large Dutch oven, mix together the sliced green onions (discard the green hollow parts), hash browns, broth and seasoning. Cook over medium-high heat while stirring occasionally.
2. Once the ingredients reach a low boil, reduce the heat to medium-low and then cover the Dutch oven and simmer for 10 minutes and remember to stir occasionally.
3. Once the potatoes are done, puree using an immersion blender; the soup should be nice and thick.
4. Add the cheddar and stir until combined.
5. Remove from the heat and serve while warm. You can garnish with the green parts of the onions and extra cheddar if you wish.

Nutrition: Calories 386 Fat 11g, Carbs 34g, Protein 13g

83. CAULIFLOWER SOUP

PREPARATION: 10 MIN **COOKING:** 35 MIN **SERVINGS:** 5

INGREDIENTS

- 2-3 cups vegetable broth
- 1 tablespoon chopped fresh rosemary (or 1 teaspoon dried rosemary)
- 1/2 head of cauliflower, roughly chopped
- 3-4 cloves garlic, smashed
- 1 yellow onion, roughly chopped

DIRECTIONS

1. In a Dutch oven over medium heat, heat one tablespoon of butter. Add the onion, garlic and a pinch of salt and cook for 10-12 minutes ensuring that you stir occasionally.
2. Once the onions and garlic start to brown, add the rosemary and cauliflower, increase the heat and cook for 3-5 minutes more.
3. Add the vegetable broth ensuring that it is just enough to cover the veggies. Bring the ingredients to a boil and then lower the heat.
4. Simmer for about 5 minutes, remove from heat and blend for a smoother consistency.
5. Serve hot.

Nutrition: Calories 298, Fat 9g, Carbs 15 g, Protein 12g

84. MISO SOUP

PREPARATION: 10 MIN **COOKING:** 15 MIN **SERVINGS:** 5

INGREDIENTS

- 2-3 scallions, chopped
- 1 tablespoon mellow white miso
- 4 oz tofu, chopped into bite-size pieces
- 1 heaping cup frozen mixed vegetables (such as carrots and broccoli)
- 3 cups water

Nutrition: Calories 186, Fat 6g, Carbs 13g, Protein 4g

DIRECTIONS

1. Add the water, tofu and vegetables into a large Dutch oven and then bring the ingredients to a boil.
2. Once done, reduce the heat to medium and cook for 2-3 minutes.
3. In the meantime, combine the miso and a few tablespoons of water until dissolved.
4. Remove the Dutch oven from the heat and let the soup cool for 1 minute. Add the miso mixture and stir to combine.
5. Top with scallions and serve.

85. TOMATO TORTELLINI SOUP

PREPARATION: 10 MIN **COOKING:** 15 MIN **SERVINGS:** 5

INGREDIENTS

- 1 10 oz. bag of fresh tortellini
- 1 (28 oz.) can diced fire roasted tomatoes (with liquid)
- 4 cups chicken stock

Nutrition: Calories 347, Fat 14g, Carbs 21g, Protein 9g

DIRECTIONS

1. In a Dutch oven over medium-high heat, add the fire roasted tomatoes and chicken stock, allow the ingredients to come to a roaring boil.
2. Once boiling, turn off the heat and use an immersion blender to purée the soup.
3. Add fresh tortellini and cook for 3-4 minutes more.
4. Remove and serve hot.

86. BROCCOLI CHEESE SOUP

PREPARATION: 10 MIN **COOKING:** 25 MIN **SERVINGS:** 5

INGREDIENTS

- 3 cups cheddar cheese
- 1 cup heavy cream
- 3 1/2 cups chicken broth (or vegetable broth, or bone broth)
- 4 cloves garlic (minced)
- 4 cups broccoli (cut into florets)

Nutrition: Calories 344, Fat 22 g, Carbs 18g, Protein 7g

DIRECTIONS

1. In a large Dutch oven over medium heat, add some oil and sauté the garlic for 1 minute or until fragrant.
2. Add the heavy cream, chopped broccoli and chicken broth. Increase the heat and bring the ingredients to a boil. Once boiling, reduce the heat and then simmer for 10-20 minutes; the broccoli should be tender.
3. Gradually stir in the shredded cheddar cheese, and stir until melted. You can start by adding 1/2 cup of cheese and wait until it melts before repeating until all the cheese is used up. Remember to keep the heat low.
4. Remove and serve immediately.

FISH AND SEAFOOD RECIPES

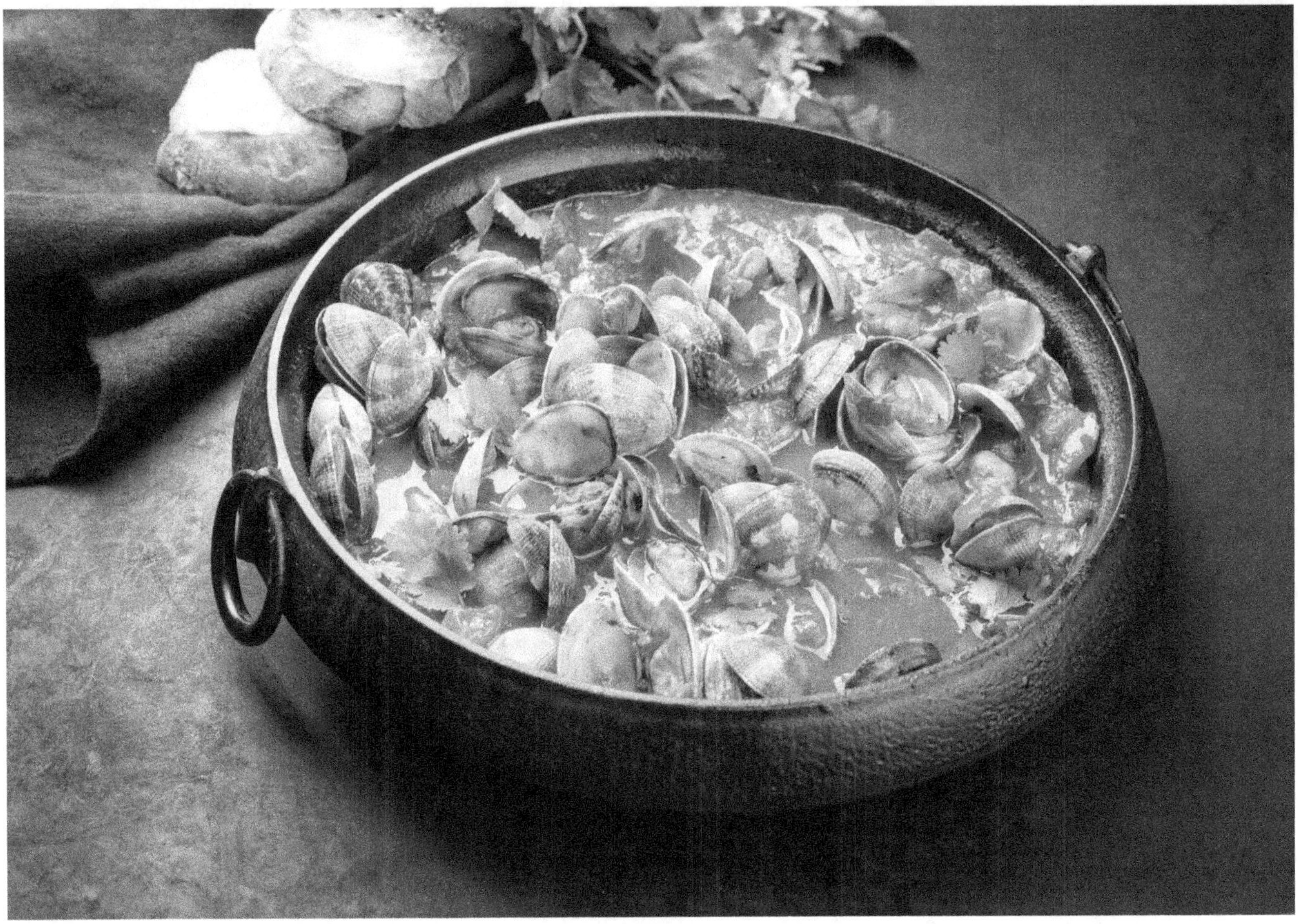

87. TILAPIA WITH CHIVE BLESSING

PREPARATION: 5 MIN **COOKING:** 30 MIN **SERVINGS:** 4

INGREDIENTS

- 4 tilapia fillets, approximately 6 oz each
- 1 tablespoon butter
- ½ cup plain Greek yogurt
- ¼ cup fresh chives, chopped
- 1 tablespoon lemon zest

DIRECTIONS

1. Preheat broiler.
2. Brush the tilapia fillets with butter and season with salt and pepper. Place fish fillets in a baking dish and put under the broiler for approximately 6-7 minutes, or until cooked through.
3. In a blender, combine the Greek yogurt, chives, and lemon zest. Blend until creamy and smooth.
4. Transfer tilapia fillets to serving plates and garnish with a drizzle of the creamy chive sauce.
5. Serve immediately with remaining sauce on the side.

Nutrition: Calories 392, Fat 23 g, Carbs 22.3 g, Protein 24.7 g

88. PASTA WITH CLAMS AND PANCETTA

PREPARATION: 15 MIN **COOKING:** 50 MIN **SERVINGS:** 4

INGREDIENTS

- 2 oz. pancetta, thinly sliced and chopped
- ¾ teaspoon red pepper flakes, crushed
- 1 (28 oz.) can whole tomatoes, peeled and crushed
- 4 oz. (about 1 cup) ditalini pasta or other short cut pasta
- A handful of torn basil leaves (optional)

DIRECTIONS

1. Add the oil to the Dutch oven and heat it over medium heat.
2. Add the pancetta and stir-cook for 4–5 minutes until it begins to crisp.
3. Add the onion and stir cook for 6–8 minutes until softened.
4. Add the garlic and stir cook for 4–5 minutes until fragrant.
5. Mix in the red pepper flakes.
6. Add the crushed tomatoes.
7. Over medium-high heat, simmer and cook for 12–15 minutes until liquid is reduced to half.
8. Add the water and clams. Cover and simmer over low heat for 8–10 minutes.
9. Uncover and remove the opened clams.
10. Cover again and cook the remaining clams for 15 more minutes. Discard any unopened ones; remove the opened clams.
11. Add the pasta and cook for 8–10 minutes until al dente.
12. Mix the clams back into the Dutch oven. Add the fresh basil if desired.
13. Serve warm.

Nutrition: Calories 407, Fat 16 g, Carbs 35 g, Protein 30 g

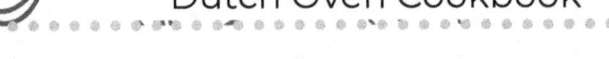

Dutch Oven Cookbook

89. BEER MUSTARD SHRIMP

PREPARATION: 15 MIN   **COOKING:** 30 MIN   **SERVINGS:** 4

INGREDIENTS

- 1 cup whole-wheat pastry flour or all-purpose flour
- 1 teaspoon Dijon mustard
- 1 cup pale ale or light-colored beer
- 1 lb. (13–15 pieces) raw shrimp, peeled and deveined, tails left on
- Pepper to taste

Nutrition: Calories 173, Fat 8.5 g, Carbs 6.5 g, Protein 16 g

DIRECTIONS

1. Add the flour, mustard, beer, and ¼ teaspoon of the salt to a mixing bowl. Mix well to make a smooth batter.
2. Cook shrimp in two batches.
3. Dip the shrimp in the batter, holding them by their tails.
4. Add the shrimp one at a time and stir-cook for 3–4 minutes until evenly brown. Drain over paper towels.
5. Repeat with the remaining 1 tablespoon of oil and the other half of the shrimp.
6. Serve warm.

90. TILAPIA NUGGETS

PREPARATION: 15 MIN   **COOKING:** 10 MIN   **SERVINGS:** 4

INGREDIENTS

- 1½ cups all-purpose flour
- 2 lbs. tilapia fillets, cut into bite-sized chunks
- 2 cups dry pancake mix
- 1-pint club soda
- 2 cups of vegetable oil
- Tartar sauce to taste

Nutrition: Calories 308, Fat 3 g, Carbs 42 g, Protein 28 g

DIRECTIONS

1. Add the flour to a bowl. Coat the fish chunks with flour. Place them over paper towels and set aside for 5 minutes.
2. Coat the fish chunks with the batter.
3. Add the oil to the Dutch oven and heat it to 400°F.
4. Add the coated fish chunks and fry for 3 minutes per side until evenly brown.
5. Drain over paper towels and serve warm.

91. BAKED SALMON WITH HERBS

PREPARATION: 15 MIN   **COOKING:** 35 MIN   **SERVINGS:** 4

INGREDIENTS

- 2 tablespoons butter
- 1 lemon, sliced
- 2 bunches of dill
- 2 lbs. salmon fillet
- ¾ cup white wine
- Salt and pepper to taste

Nutrition: Calories 405, Fat 21.1 g, Carbs 3.4 g, Protein 44.5 g

DIRECTIONS

1. Arrange the lemon slices on the bottom of the Dutch oven.
2. Arrange the dill on top of the lemon and place the salmon fillet on top of that.
3. Pour in the white wine and season with salt and pepper.
4. Cover and cook at 350°F for about 10 minutes.
5. Remove the lid and continue cooking for another 20–25 minutes.

92. BAKED TROUT WITH CHERRY TOMATOES

PREPARATION: 15 MIN   **COOKING:** 45 MIN   **SERVINGS:** 4

INGREDIENTS

- 2 tablespoons butter
- 2 tablespoons butter
- 1 lb. potatoes, sliced
- 1 lb. cherry tomatoes
- 2 lbs. whole trout

DIRECTIONS

1. Coat the Dutch oven with butter.
2. Arrange the potato slices and cherry tomatoes in the Dutch oven and season with salt and pepper.
3. Bake at 350°F for about 20 minutes.
4. Place the trout on top of the potatoes and cherry tomatoes and drizzle some butter on top of the fish.
5. Cover and bake for about 20 minutes more.
6. Remove the lid and cook for another 10 minutes.

Nutrition: Calories 597, Fat 29.5 g, Carbs 23.6 g, Protein 58.2 g

93. TILAPIA CACCIATORE

PREPARATION: 15 MIN   **COOKING:** 30 MIN   **SERVINGS:** 4

INGREDIENTS

- 2 tablespoons butter
- 2 lbs. tilapia fillets
- 2 cups tomato sauce
- ¼ cup white wine
- ¾ cup diced Kalamata olives

DIRECTIONS

1. Warm the butter in the Dutch oven over medium heat.
2. Season the fish fillets with salt and pepper. Add them to the heated oil and cook for about 5 minutes on each side.
3. Pour in the white wine and cook uncovered for about 5 minutes.
4. When half of the wine has evaporated, pour in the tomato sauce
5. Stir in the diced Kalamata olives and cook, covered, for 15–20 minutes.
6. When the tomato sauce has thickened and the fish is cooked, serve on plates.

Nutrition: Calories 302, Fat 10.5 g, Carbs 7.7 g, Protein 43.8 g

94. SEAFOOD RISOTTO

PREPARATION: 15 MIN   **COOKING:** 40 MIN   **SERVINGS:** 4

INGREDIENTS

- 1 onion, diced finely
- ½ lb. frozen seafood mix
- 1½ cups arborio rice
- ½ cup white wine
- 1-quart water

DIRECTIONS

1. Warm the butter and butter in the Dutch oven over medium heat.
2. Stir in the onion and cook for about 5 minutes or until tender.
3. Stir in the seafood mix and cook for about 5 minutes.
4. Stir in the rice and cook for 5 more minutes.
5. While stirring constantly, pour in the water, ½ cup at a time, mixing well so the mixture remains creamy but not too watery.
6. The risotto is done when the rice is cooked through.
7. Serve while it's still creamy with a dash of pepper on top.

Nutrition: Calories 457, Fat 13.7g, Carbs 62.1g, Protein 13.3 g

95. CALAMARI FRA DIAVOLO

PREPARATION: 15 MIN   **COOKING:** 40 MIN   **SERVINGS:** 4

INGREDIENTS

- 2 tablespoons butter
- 2 lbs. fresh squid, cut into rings
- ½ cup red wine
- 1 (28 oz.) can tomato sauce
- 2 teaspoons chili flakes

DIRECTIONS

1. Warm the butter and butter in the Dutch oven over medium heat.
2. Stir in the squid rings and cook for about 5 minutes.
3. Pour in the wine, water, and tomato sauce.
4. Cover and cook for 30 minutes.
5. When the mixture is almost thick and most of the liquid has evaporated, serve alone or on top of pasta or crusty bread.

Nutrition: Calories 344, Fat 10.5 g, Carbs 19.3 g, Protein 38.1 g

96. SEAFOOD STEW

PREPARATION: 15 MIN   **COOKING:** 40 MIN   **SERVINGS:** 4

INGREDIENTS

- 2 tablespoons butter
- 1 medium onion, diced
- 3 cloves garlic, minced
- 1 (14 oz.) bag of frozen vegetables
- 2 lbs. seafood mix

DIRECTIONS

1. Warm the butter in the Dutch oven over medium heat.
2. Cook the diced onion and garlic for about 5 minutes until tender.
3. Stir in the frozen veggies and seafood and cook for 10 minutes.
4. Pour in the water and cook for 30 minutes.
5. Serve with bread if desired.

Nutrition: Calories 348, Fat 9.3 g, Carbs 22.9 g, Protein 36 g

97. CAJUN SCALLOPS

PREPARATION: 5 MIN   **COOKING:** 10 MIN   **SERVINGS:** 4

INGREDIENTS

- 1-lb. fresh scallops
- 2 teaspoons Cajun seasoning
- 2 tablespoons butter, melted
- 2 cups fresh spinach
- 1 teaspoon crushed red pepper flakes

DIRECTIONS

1. Begin by liberally sprinkling the scallops with the Cajun seasoning.
2. Add butter to a large skillet and heat over medium. Add the spinach. Cook until spinach is wilted, approximately 1-2 minutes.
3. Add the scallops and cook for one minute, or until browned on one side. Turn and cook an additional 3-4 minutes, or until cooked through.
4. Remove from heat and serve immediately.

Nutrition: Calories 192, Fat 23 g, Carbs 22.3 g, Protein 24.7 g

98. SORT OF SALMON NIÇOISE

PREPARATION: 10 MIN **COOKING:** 30 MIN **SERVINGS:** 3

INGREDIENTS

- 2 x 4 oz. gram salmon fillets
- 2 heaped tablespoons Greek yogurt
- 100 oz. green beans
- 2 large free-range eggs
- 8 black olives

Nutrition: Calories 374, Fat 13g, Carbs 32g, Protein 39g

DIRECTIONS

1. Place the salmon skin-side down to steam for 8 minutes in a colander over a Dutch oven of boiling salted water.
2. Line the beans, trim just the stem's end, then boil for 6 minutes in the water under the salmon, or just fried, but not squeaky. Drop gently in the eggs to cook side by side for precisely about 5 minutes.
3. In the meantime, crush the olives and slice the flesh finely. Add sea salt and black pepper, blend half of the olives through the yogurt with a splash of Red wine vinegar, which should be appropriately flavored.
4. Move the salmon to a board and remove in the colander the eggs and beans.
5. In the dressing, throw the beans and break between your bowls. Cool enough to handle, refresh the eggs under cold water, then peel and cut into quarters.
6. Flake over the salmon, remove the meat, cover the eggs and blot the rest of the chopped olives.
7. Finish with 1 tablespoon of extra virgin butter and a small pinch of pepper.

99. SEARED SALMON WITH CAPER SAUCE

PREPARATION: 15 MIN **COOKING:** 30 MIN **SERVINGS:** 4

INGREDIENTS

- 4 salmon fillets, approximately 6 oz. each
- 2 tablespoon butter
- 2 tablespoons capers
- 1 cup white wine
- 1 tablespoon Dijon mustard

Nutrition: Calories 292, Fat 23 g, Carbs 22.3 g, Protein 24.7 g

DIRECTIONS

1. Brush the salmon with butter
2. Warm a skillet over medium-high heat. Add the salmon and cook for three minutes. Reduce heat to medium, turn the salmon and cook for an additional 5 minutes. Remove from pan and set aside.
3. Add the capers, white wine, and Dijon mustard into the skillet. Bring to a slow boil while stirring constantly. Reduce heat and simmer for 5-7 minutes.
4. Add salmon back into pan and heat with sauce for 3-4 minutes.
5. Transfer salmon to serving plates and top with caper sauce before serving.

100. FOIL PACK GRILLED LEMONY SALMON WITH ASPARAGUS

PREPARATION: 20 MIN **COOKING:** 12 MIN **SERVINGS:** 5

INGREDIENTS

- 20 asparagus spears, trimmed
- 4 (6 oz.) skin-on salmon fillets
- 2 tablespoons melted butter, divided
- ¼ cup fresh dill, to garnish
- ¼ cup fresh cilantro, to garnish

DIRECTIONS

1. Place 4 large pieces of foil on a flat surface, and arrange 5 pieces of asparagus on each piece. Top each one with a fillet of fish.
2. Brush butter on each fillet, and then season them with salt and pepper.
3. Place slices of lemon on top.
4. Loosely wrap the fillets to make packets.
5. Heat the grill on high, and place the foil packets on the grill.
6. Cook for about 12 minutes.
7. Garnish with cilantro and dill, and enjoy!

Nutrition: Calories 359, Fat 18.1 g, Carbs 0.7 g, Protein 44.5 g

101. CREAMY HERBED SHRIMP PASTA

PREPARATION: 15 MIN **COOKING:** 15 MIN **SERVINGS:** 4

INGREDIENTS

- 1 lb. dried angel hair pasta
- 1 lb. medium-sized shrimp, cleaned and deveined
- ½ cup butter
- 2 cups fresh herb mix (prepackaged or your choice of basil, parsley, mint, etc.)
- ½ cup fresh grated parmesan cheese

DIRECTIONS

1. Bring a large pot of water to boil and cook angel hair according to package instructions.
2. In a blender or food processor combine the herb mix and parmesan cheese. Blend or pulse until combined. Slowly add in all but one tablespoon of the butter, blending until smooth. Set aside.
3. Heat the remaining butter in a sauté pan. Add the shrimp and season with salt and pepper. Cook over medium heat for 5-6 minutes, or until shrimp is cooked through.
4. Add the angel hair pasta and ¼ cup of the pasta water to the pan with the shrimp and toss.
5. Add the pesto sauce to the pasta, tossing well until pasta and shrimp are evenly coated.
6. Serve immediately.

Nutrition: Calories 312, Fat 23 g, Carbs 22.3 g, Protein 24.7 g, Sodium 877 mg

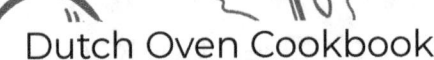

102. KISSED BY AN ITALIAN WHITEFISH

PREPARATION: 10 MIN   **COOKING:** 15 MIN   **SERVINGS:** 4

INGREDIENTS

- 4 whitefish fillets, approximately 5-6 oz each
- 1 cup fresh grated parmesan cheese
- ¼ cup fresh parsley
- 2 cloves garlic, crushed and minced
- 1 lemon, quartered

Nutrition: Calories 332, Fat 23 g, Carbs 22.3 g, Protein 24.7 g

DIRECTIONS

1. Preheat oven to 400°F.
2. Season the whitefish with salt and pepper.
3. In a bowl, combine the parmesan cheese, parsley, and minced garlic. Mix well.
4. Pat both sides of the fish with parmesan mixture, creating a thick coat. Place fish in a baking dish.
5. Place the fish in the oven and bake for 12-15 minutes, or until done.
6. Garnish with lemon wedges before serving.

103. FRESH AND SIMPLE FISH TACOS

PREPARATION: 5 MIN   **COOKING:** 10 MIN   **SERVINGS:** 4

INGREDIENTS

- 1 lb. tilapia, or other mild fish, cut into cubes
- ¼ cup fresh cilantro, chopped
- ½ cup fresh pico de gallo
- 1 cup red cabbage, shredded
- 1 tablespoon butter

Nutrition: Calories 392, Fat 23 g, Carbs 22.3 g, Protein 24.7 g

DIRECTIONS

1. Preheat the broiler.
2. Drizzle tilapia with butter and season with salt and pepper.
3. Place under the broiler and cook for approximately 7 minutes, or until flakey and cooked through.
4. Layer the fish on warmed tortillas, with cabbage and pico de gallo. Garnish with cilantro. Serve immediately.

104. LEMON SHRIMP AND PASTA

PREPARATION: 5 MIN   **COOKING:** 15 MIN   **SERVINGS:** 4

INGREDIENTS

- 1 lb. dried linguine
- 1 lb. shrimp, cleaned and deveined
- 1 tablespoon lemon infused butter
- 1 cup fresh snow peas, shelled
- Fresh shaved asiago cheese for garnish

Nutrition: Calories 392, Fat 23 g, Carbs 22.3 g, Protein 24.7 g

DIRECTIONS

1. Prepare and boil a large pot of water. Cook linguine according to package instructions. After draining the pasta, dress with 1 tablespoon of the lemon butter
2. Add 1 tablespoon of the lemon butter to a sauté pan and heat over medium. Add the shrimp and cook for 3 minutes before turning over.
3. Add the peas and season with salt and pepper. Cook for an additional 3-4 minutes, or until shrimp is cooked through.
4. Place the pasta onto serving plates and top with shrimp and peas. Garnish with fresh shaved asiago before serving.

105. LEMON BUTTER SALMON FOIL PACKS

PREPARATION: 20 MIN **COOKING:** 10 MIN **SERVINGS:** 5

INGREDIENTS

- 2 lemons or limes, thinly sliced
- 6–8 salmon fillets
- 4 tablespoons butter, divided
- ½ cup white wine

Nutrition: Calories 338, Fat 18 g, Carbs 5 g, Protein 35 g

DIRECTIONS

1. Preheat the grill to medium heat, and prepare 4 large pieces of foil with cooking spray.
2. Place one large piece of foil on a flat surface.
3. Season with salt and pepper, and layer on some lime or lemon slices.
4. Top with salmon fillets, and season with more salt if desired.
5. Place a pat of butter on the fish, and top it with a splash of wine.
6. Fold the foil in half and then fold up the edges to seal the packet.
7. Repeat with the other servings.
8. Grill for 12 minutes, until the fish flakes easily with a fork.

106. FISH TACOS

PREPARATION: 10 MIN **COOKING:** 20 MIN **SERVINGS:** 5

INGREDIENTS

- 1 tablespoon butter
- 8 oz. salmon pieces or fillets
- 2 corn or flour tortillas
- 1 cup fresh salsa
- ½ cup romaine lettuce, sliced

Nutrition: Calories 392, Fat 23 g, Carbs 22.3 g, Protein 24.7 g

DIRECTIONS

1. Place a rack over the campfire, and heat a pan.
2. Melt the butter, and cook the salmon for 5–7 minutes on each side, until it is cooked through. Set it aside.
3. Warm the corn tortillas on both sides in the same pan.
4. Place the salmon pieces on the tortillas, and top with a generous amount of salsa, lettuce,
5. Serve and enjoy.

107. FOIL PACKED HONEY-LIME TILAPIA AND CORN

PREPARATION: 20 MIN **COOKING:** 15 MIN **SERVINGS:** 5

INGREDIENTS

- 5 tilapia fillets
- 2 tablespoons honey
- 3 limes, sliced
- 3 ears corn, shucked
- ¼ cup butter

Nutrition: Calories 343, Fat 13.2 g, Carbs 28.6 g, Protein 35.3 g

DIRECTIONS

1. Cut foil into 5 pieces, 10–12 inches long, and heat the grill.
2. Top each piece of foil with a fillet, and brush it with honey.
3. Top the fish with lime and corn kernels, and sprinkle cilantro on top.
4. Fold and seal the packets, and grill for about 15 minutes.
5. Serve when the fish is cooked through.

108. CILANTRO-LIME SHRIMP FOIL PACKS

PREPARATION: 20 MIN   **COOKING:** 10 MIN   **SERVINGS:** 4

INGREDIENTS

- 1 lb. medium shrimp, peeled and deveined
- 4 ears corn, quartered
- 4 cloves garlic, minced
- 2 tablespoons freshly chopped cilantro
- 2 tablespoons butter

Nutrition: Calories 336, Fat 12.5 g, Carbs 33.6 g, Protein 29.8 g

DIRECTIONS

1. In a large bowl, combine the shrimp, corn.
2. Toss well to combine all the ingredients.
3. Take four pieces of foil and divide the shrimp mixture onto each. Dot each with butter, and divide the lime slices over the top.
4. Seal the packets.
5. Heat a grill and place the packets on it. Grill for about 10 minutes.
6. Serve when the shrimp is pink and cooked through.

109. FISH AND VEGETABLES ON A SKEWER

PREPARATION: 20 MIN   **COOKING:** 10 MIN   **SERVINGS:** 5

INGREDIENTS

- ⅓ cup orange juice
- 4–6 oz. salmon, cut into small pieces
- 1 small zucchini, cut into chunks
- 1 cup cherry tomatoes
- 1 large green or yellow bell pepper, diced

Nutrition: Calories 121, Fat 4 g, Carbs 9 g, Protein 14 g

DIRECTIONS

1. Oil and preheat a grill over medium heat.
2. Combine the orange juice in a bowl and add all the remaining ingredients. Let it sit for 10 minutes.
3. Skewer the fish pieces, alternating with the zucchini, cherry tomatoes, and bell pepper.
4. Grill the skewers for 5 minutes per side, or until the salmon is cooked and the vegetables are tender.

110. GARLIC SHRIMP

PREPARATION: 15 MIN   **COOKING:** 10 MIN   **SERVINGS:** 5

INGREDIENTS

- 1 lemon, juice only
- ½ stick butter, melted
- 1 cup parsley, chopped
- 4 cloves garlic, minced
- 1 lb. unpeeled shrimp

Nutrition: Calories 412, Fat 23.5 g, Carbs 7.4 g, Protein 39 g

DIRECTIONS

1. In a mixing bowl or resealable bag, combine all the ingredients EXCEPT the shrimp, and mix well.
2. Add the shrimp, and stir to coat.
3. Set out two pieces of aluminum foil, and place half the shrimp mixture on each.
4. Fold the foils into packets and seal them well.
5. Grill over high heat for about 10 minutes.
6. Serve hot.

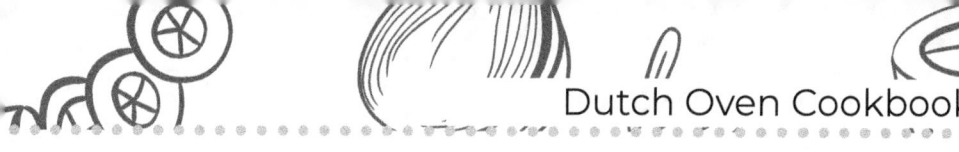

111. DUTCH OVEN-BAKED SALMON

PREPARATION: 10 MIN **COOKING:** 50 MIN **SERVINGS:** 4

INGREDIENTS

- 1 lb. of salmon skinned on 1 side or four salmon fillets
- 3-tablespoonful Dijon mustard
- 16 crackers, crushed
- Dill weed

Nutrition: Calories 498, Fat 15g, Carbs 28g, Protein 33g

DIRECTIONS

1. Using a non-stick cooking spray, spray the Dutch oven with the spray. Place the salmon fillet in the equipped Dutch oven, skinned side down.
2. Spread the mustard generously over the fish and then sprinkle with crushed cracker crumbs.
3. Add a little dill weed at your leisure or lemon pepper, depending on your choice. Allow it to bake at 350 degrees for approximately 15-20 minutes.

112. BEER ME-LIGHTLY FRIED FISH FILLETS

PREPARATION: 10 MIN **COOKING:** 35 MIN **SERVINGS:** 3

INGREDIENTS

- 1 lb. Fish Fillets
- 1 Cup Buttermilk Pancake Mix
- 1 Cup Beer
- 1 Cup Flour

Nutrition: Calories 398, Fat 12g, Carbs 32g, Protein 28g

DIRECTIONS

1. When cooking Fish Fillets, the oil has to be beautiful and hot too, so we should heat it in the Dutch oven.
2. Clean and dry the Fish Fillets.
3. Dredge the Fish Fillets in the flour. All we want is just flour covering all over the water.
4. Mix the Pancake mix with about three-quarter Cup of beer. To make it smooth, mix it with a fork. Take the Fish Fillets floured and dip them in the Batter. Finally, we want a coating that is even.
5. Place the Fish Fillets in the oil and cook until Golden, Brown, and Delicious are outside. The inside should be fresh, moist and shiny once the outside is dry. Just cook 2 at a time when frying is a significant no-no while overcrowding the pot.
6. Once they're all done, let them drain a little on a paper towel.
7. You can sprinkle on them after that a little dill, pepper, or lemon, but that's not required.

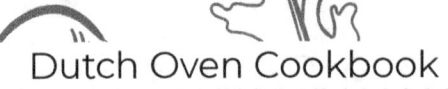

BEEF

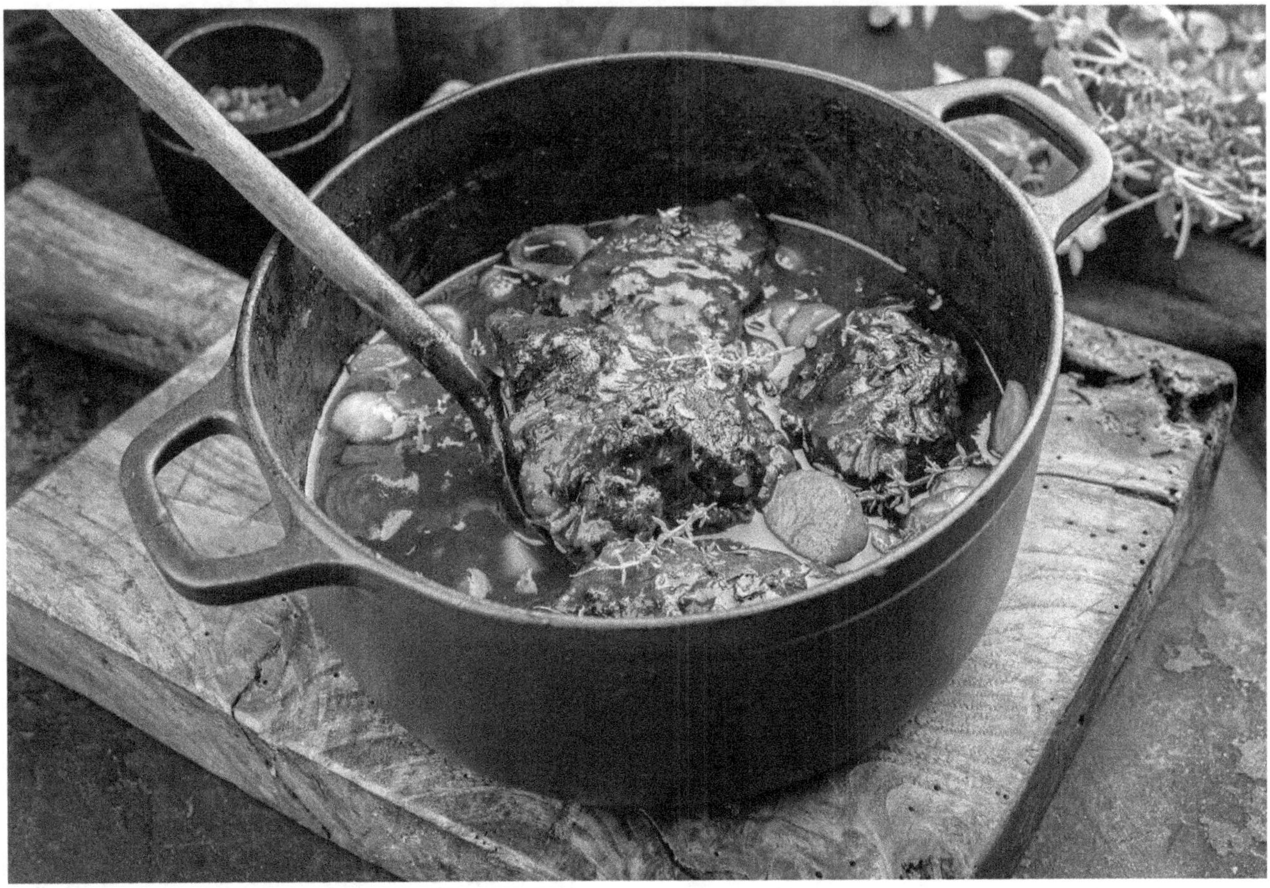

113. ITALIAN SEARED BEEF

PREPARATION: 10 MIN **COOKING:** 40 MIN **SERVINGS:** 3

INGREDIENTS

- 1 tablespoon pine nuts
- 9 oz. rump steak
- 2 heaped teaspoons green pesto
- 1.5 oz. rocket
- ½ oz. Parmesan cheese

DIRECTIONS

1. Put your Dutch oven on high heat, toasting the pine nuts as it heats up, tossing regularly and removing when golden.
2. Cut the fat off the rump, chop the fat thinly, put it in the pan to make and crisp while cutting the sinew off the backside, and then season it with salt and black pepper.
3. Place with a rolling pin between 2 sheets of greaseproof paper and tenderize the meat to 1 cm thick.
4. Excavate and save the crispy bits of fat, then sear the steak on each side in the hot pan for 1 minute, until it blushes in the center. Take off to aside.
5. Spread the pesto over a plate for sharing. Slice the steak thinly at an angle, then flatten the steak. Place the rocket on top, scatter, if you like, over the pine nuts and crispy fat reserved.
6. Mix with a tbsp. of extra virgin butter and drizzle over the steak resting juices. Shave over the Parmesan and toss before serving.

Nutrition: Calories 458, Fat 18g, Carbs 19g, Protein 52g

114. GROUND BEEF SKEWERS

PREPARATION: 20 MIN **COOKING:** 20 MIN **SERVINGS:** 3

INGREDIENTS

- 1 lb. ground beef
- 3 cloves garlic, minced
- 2 green onions, minced
- 1 teaspoon fresh ginger, minced
- 1 cup red onion, minced

DIRECTIONS

1. At home, combine all the ingredients seal the mixture in a plastic container or a sturdy bag.
2. At the campsite, oil and preheat the grill or start the campfire.
3. Separate the meat mixture into six pieces, and form each into a cylinder shape. Pierce with skewers.
4. Grill over an open flame, until browned and cooked through.
5. Serve.

Nutrition: Calories 227, Fat 15.3 g, Carbs 8.6 g, Protein 14.3 g

115. BEEF & POTATO PACKETS

PREPARATION: 30 MIN **COOKING:** 25 MIN **SERVINGS:** 5

INGREDIENTS

- 1 tablespoon butter
- 2 tablespoons sherry vinegar
- 1 medium sweet potato, peeled and thinly sliced
- ½ cup onion, sliced
- 4 (6 oz.) servings of beef steak, trimmed of fat

Nutrition: Calories 566, Fat 41 g, Carbs 12.7 g, Protein 34.2 g

DIRECTIONS

1. Combine the oil, sherry vinegar, sweet potato, and onion in a bowl. Let it sit for few minutes.
2. Lay out four double-layer sheets of foil, and coat the foil with cooking spray.
3. Using a slotted spoon, remove the vegetables from the sauce, and arrange them on the four foil pieces.
4. Place the meat in the sauce, and turn it to coat.
5. Top each serving with a piece of steak, and pour the sauce over.
6. Seal the packets, and place them on the grill.
7. Cook for 25 minutes, turning halfway.
8. Check that the steak is cooked to your liking, and serve.

116. ANN'S BRISKET

PREPARATION: 10 MIN **COOKING:** 20 MIN **SERVINGS:** 3

INGREDIENTS

- 3-4 lb. beef brisket
- 2-3 tbsp. flour
- Seasoned tenderizer

Nutrition: Calories 409, Fat 22g, Carbs 21g, Protein 47g

DIRECTIONS

1. Tenderizer coat brisket well. Wrap with 2 heavy-duty foil covers. Chill overnight. Cover and cook for about 7 hours in the Dutch oven. You can cook it more quickly, but it's slowly cooked juicier.
2. Remove the foil and put it on a warm serving plate. Create a thin gravy with milk, rice. Before serving, pour over the brisket.

117. SWISS STEAK

PREPARATION: 10 MIN **COOKING:** 40 MIN **SERVINGS:** 3

INGREDIENTS

- 3 lb. round steak
- 3 stalks celery, peeled, chopped fine
- 3 tbsp.. butter
- 1/2 c catsup (optional)
- 1 tbsp. chopped parsley

DIRECTIONS

1. In your Dutch oven, brown steak in butter. Add parsley, celery, and catsup. Cover and cook 2-1/2 hours. If the mixture thickens too much, 1/2 cup water may be required.

Nutrition: Calories 648, Fat 32g, Carbs 10g, Protein 56g

118. ONION SWISS STEAK

PREPARATION: 10 MIN   **COOKING:** 120 MIN   **SERVINGS:** 3

INGREDIENTS

- 2 pkg onion soup mix
- 3 lb. round steak, 3/4" thick
- 2 cans (10 oz.) tomatoes

DIRECTIONS

1. Cut the steak into servings, and place in the Dutch oven. Sprinkle the soup of the onion over the top and pour over the tomatoes. Cover and cook for 2 to 3 hours over a slow fire or until meat is finished and tender.

Nutrition: Calories 678, Fat 34g, Carbs 11g, Protein 58g

119. POOR MAN'S STEAK

PREPARATION: 10 MIN   **COOKING:** 60 MIN   **SERVINGS:** 3

INGREDIENTS

- 2 cans Mushroom Soup
- 2 lb. pkg Ground beef
- 2 tsp. Salt
- 1 1/3 c Milk
- Margarine

DIRECTIONS

1. Mix meat, salt, and milk together. Pack in pans of the loaf. Let stand overnight or for at least 6 hours in the refrigerator. Cut into slices and margarine brown. In the Dutch oven, mix the soup with 1 cup of water and pour over the beef. Bake 1-1/2 hours at 350°F.

Nutrition: Calories 432, Fat 19g, Carbs 9g, Protein 38g

120. CORNED BEEF & CABBAGE

PREPARATION: 10 MIN   **COOKING:** 120 MIN   **SERVINGS:** 3

INGREDIENTS

- 2 lb. well-trimmed corned beef
- 1 small onion, quartered
- 1 little head green cabbage and cut into six wedges
- Six medium carrots cut into quarters

DIRECTIONS

1. In the Dutch oven, pour enough cold water on corned beef to cover. Stir in the onion. Heat to simmer, then lower. Cover and cook till around 2 hours until the beef is tender. Remove the beef and keep it warm. Skim broth fat. Heat to boil, add cabbage and carrots. Reduce heat and cook for 15 minutes.

Nutrition: Calories 468, Fat 11g, Carbs 11g, Protein 39g

121. SAUSAGE BALLS

PREPARATION: 10 MIN **COOKING:** 15 MIN **SERVINGS:** 3

INGREDIENTS

- 1 Egg
- 3 Bisquick
- 6 oz. Grated Cheddar Cheese
- 1 lb. Sausage (mild or hot)

DIRECTIONS

1. Combine all the ingredients. Mix with your hands the best. Pinch off small pieces and mold them into balls.
2. Bake at 350°F in Dutch oven for 10-15 minutes.

Nutrition: Calories 418, Fat 21g, Carbs 19g, Protein 27g

122. GREAT BEEF STEW

PREPARATION: 10 MIN **COOKING:** 30 MIN **SERVINGS:** 3

INGREDIENTS

- 1/4 lb. chuck steak
- 5 lbs. of potatoes
- 5 lbs. of carrots

DIRECTIONS

1. Let the beef cook at a full boil for 30 minutes, throw in carrots + potatoes, bring to boil, and serve once the carrots and potatoes are tender.

Nutrition: Calories 334, Fat 21g, Carbs 21g, Protein 42g

123. BEEF GOULASH

PREPARATION: 10 MIN **COOKING:** 60 MIN **SERVINGS:** 3

INGREDIENTS

- 3 lb. beef, cubed
- 1 can mushroom soup
- Water

DIRECTIONS

1. Brown the meat in your Dutch oven cooking oil. Add soup. Cover and simmer about 1 hour.

Nutrition: Calories 395, Fat 13 g, Carbs 12g, Protein 45g

124. MESS

PREPARATION: 10 MIN **COOKING:** 20 MIN **SERVINGS:** 3

INGREDIENTS

- 1 can tomato soup
- 1-1/2 lb. ground beef
- 1 can (16 oz.) French-style green beans
- 1 small onion chopped
- 1 can mushrooms

Nutrition: Calories 313, Fat 18g, Carbs 12g, Protein 37g

DIRECTIONS

1. Brown ground beef as well as onion until the onion is transparent you do that by frying in your Dutch oven. Drain and add other ingredients. Heat through for about 20 minutes and salt to taste. Serve plain or on top of spaghetti or noodles.

125. TACO PIE

PREPARATION: 10 MIN **COOKING:** 20 MIN **SERVINGS:** 3

INGREDIENTS

- 1-1/2 lb. ground beef
- 1 medium jar Taco sauce
- Four large corn tortillas
- 1 8 oz. pkg shredded cheddar cheese
- 1 can (8 oz..) tomato puree

Nutrition: Calories 349, Fat 21g, Carbs 27g, Protein 48g

DIRECTIONS

1. Brown ground beef, drain. Combine taco sauce and tomato puree. Line Dutch oven with aluminum foil.
2. Layer 2 shells of tortilla in the Dutch oven. Layer half of the ground beef on top and pour over 1/2 taco sauce. Place 2 more shells of tortilla on top and place them in the rest of the meat and pour over the rest of the taco sauce. Sprinkle the cheese with it.
3. Cover and bake until it melts the cheese. Variations Apply to meat chopped onions, mushrooms, or tomatoes.

126. BACON, BEEF, AND BEANS CASSEROLE

PREPARATION: 10 MIN **COOKING:** 45 MIN **SERVINGS:** 3

INGREDIENTS

- ¾ lb. Bacon
- 1 can of Biscuits
- ¾ lb. Ground Beef
- 20 oz. Canned Baked Beans
- ½ Cup Steak Sauce or Barbecue Sauce

Nutrition: Calories 578, Fat 20g, Carbs 32g, Protein 40g

DIRECTIONS

1. This tasty and satisfying dinner is great for cold evenings. Grill the bacon over medium heat in the Dutch oven. Remove from fire, drain and chop until finished. Cook the ground beef until it's cooked.
2. Add the Baked Beans, chopped Bacon, and Sauce to the Dutch oven. Stir until it becomes well mixed and comes to a boil. Take it off of direct fire (think low to medium heat) and layer out the Meat's biscuits with Bean mixture. Cover then cook for around 10 minutes or until the biscuits are golden, brown, and delicious.

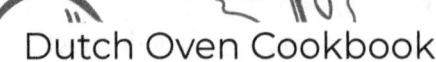
Dutch Oven Cookbook

127. SPINACH STEAK PINWHEELS

PREPARATION: 10 MIN **COOKING:** 20 MIN **SERVINGS:** 3

INGREDIENTS

- 1½ lbs. beef top sirloin steak
- 8 bacon strips, cooked and drained
- 1 package (10 oz.) frozen chopped spinach (thawed and squeezed dry)
- ¼ cup grated Parmesan cheese

Nutrition: Calories 478, Fat 21g, Carbs 23g, Protein 43g

DIRECTIONS

1. Make diagonal steak cuts at intervals of 1 inch to within half-inch of the meat bottom. Do the reductions the other way around. Pound to the thickness of half an inch. Put bacon in the middle of the beef.
2. Combine the spinach, Parmesan cheese, salt, and cayenne in a large bowl; spoon over bacon. Roll up with toothpicks and protect them. Cut six strips.
3. Grill over medium heat for 6 minutes on each side or until the meat reaches the optimal doneness (for medium-rare, 145°F should be read by a meat thermometer; medium, 160°F; well-done, 170°F). Dispose of toothpicks and serve.

128. SUNDAY ROAST BEEF AND GRAVY

PREPARATION: 10 MIN **COOKING:** 35 MIN **SERVINGS:** 3

INGREDIENTS

- ¼ cup butter
- 1 (3 to 4 lb.) bone-in rib-eye roast
- 5 cups beef stock
- ½ bottle drinking red wine, such as Malbec (optional)

Nutrition: Calories 678, Fat 31g, Carbs 21g, Protein 65g

DIRECTIONS

1. Preheat oven to 400°F.
2. In a large Dutch oven, heat butter or a roasting pan. Put the beef in a hot pan and sear on all sides until deep golden brown.
3. For medium-rare, move the pan to the oven and roast for approximately 15 minutes per pound, resulting in estimated cooking time. Move beef to a cutting board and remove the pan from the oven. Allow meat to rest, tented with foil, before carving for at least 15 minutes.
4. To make the gravy: pour off the Dutch oven excess fat and put the pan over medium heat on the stovetop. Attach shallots and cook for around 4 to 6 minutes until soft and brown. Deglaze the pot with half-filled cup of the wine, from the bottom scrap brown bits.
5. Add remaining wine, bring it to a boil, and halve it. Add stock and cook until it is reduced by about half again. Use a fine-mesh sieve to pass the gravy and return to the pan.
6. Bring back to a boil, then will heat and cook until the desired consistency is reached. Taste and change the seasoning if necessary. Carve the beef into thin slices against the grain and serve gravely.

129. BEEF AND VEGETABLE STIR FRY

PREPARATION: 10MIN **COOKING:** 35 MIN **SERVINGS:** 3

INGREDIENTS

- 1 tablespoon butter
- 1 (16 oz.) package frozen mixed vegetables
- 1 cup stir fry sauce
- 2 teaspoons cornstarch
- 2 cups cubed cooked roast beef

Nutrition: Calories 489, Fat 17g, Carbs 21g, Protein 39g

DIRECTIONS

1. Get your Dutch oven, heat the oil. Remove the frozen vegetables and remove some water when the oil is hot, then stir. Cover and cook for 3 minutes over medium heat.
2. In a small bowl, mix the stir fry sauce with the cornstarch. Pour the vegetables into the Dutch oven and mix. Then add and stir the cooked beef.
3. Replace the cover, cook the beef and vegetables at low heat for 5 to 8 minutes, occasionally stirring, till the meat is tender, while the vegetables are still crisp.

130. BALSAMIC BRAISED BEEF RIBS

PREPARATION: 10 MIN **COOKING:** 6 H **SERVINGS:** 3

INGREDIENTS

- 3 lbs. short ribs
- 7 cloves garlic, crushed
- 2 cups tomato sauce (fresh or canned)
- ¾ cup balsamic vinegar
- 1 cup fresh figs, chopped

Nutrition: Calories 459, Fat 19g, Carbs 18g, Protein 56g

DIRECTIONS

1. Take crushed garlic cloves and rub briskly over the short ribs. Cut the ribs and place them, along with any remaining garlic pieces, into a slow cooker.
2. In a small bowl, combine the tomato sauce, balsamic vinegar, and figs. Pour over the ribs and toss to coat.
3. Cook over low heat for 6-8 hours until ribs are fall off the bone tender.

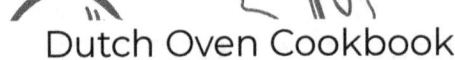
Dutch Oven Cookbook

131. GRANDMA'S WEEKEND ROAST

PREPARATION: 10 MIN **COOKING:** 125 MIN **SERVINGS:** 3

INGREDIENTS

- 1 4 lb. beef roast
- ¼ cup butter
- 3 cups yellow onion, sliced
- 3 cups beef stock
- 1 cup red wine

Nutrition: Calories 419, Fat 18g, Carbs 12g, Protein 38g

DIRECTIONS

1. Preheat oven to 325°F
2. Heat the butter in a Dutch oven over medium to medium-high heat.
3. Add the roast to the Dutch oven and brown evenly, approximately 3-5 minutes, on each side.
4. Remove meat from pan and temporarily set aside.
5. Add the onions to the pan, and cook until slightly soft, approximately 5 minutes.
6. Stir in the beef stock and red wine, and cook while stirring for 5-7 minutes. Season with additional salt and pepper, if desired.
7. Add the roast back into the Dutch oven, cover and place in the oven. Cook for 2 hours, turn roast, and then cook an additional 45 minutes.
8. Let roast rest 10 minutes before serving. Serve dressed with the tender onions and pan sauce.

132. FLANK STEAK ROULADE

PREPARATION: 10 MIN **COOKING:** 65 MIN **SERVINGS:** 3

INGREDIENTS

- 1 2 lb. flank steak, trimmed
- 1 tablespoon butter
- 3 cups fresh spinach, chopped
- 2 cups tomatoes, chopped
- 2 tablespoons prepared horseradish

Nutrition: Calories 478, Fat 13g, Carbs 11g, Protein 56g

DIRECTIONS

1. Preheat oven to 425°F
2. Heat the butter over medium heat in a sauté pan. Add the spinach and tomatoes. Cook until spinach is wilted and tomatoes have begun to release a good amount of juice, approximately 4-5 minutes. Remove from heat.
3. Add one tablespoon of the horseradish to the spinach mixture. Mix well and set aside.
4. Using a mallet, pound steak until it is approximately ¼-inch thick.
5. Take any butter that remains in the sauté pan and drizzle over the steak. Season with the remaining horseradish, salt, and pepper. Rub the mixture into the steak before turning the meat over.
6. Spread the spinach mixture along the steak. Starting at one end, begin rolling the steak lengthwise to create a pinwheel. Secure the pinwheel with several pieces of chef's twine.
7. Place the roll into a baking pan and bake for 45-50 minutes.
8. Let rest for 10 minutes before removing twine and slicing into pieces 1½-inch thick for serving.

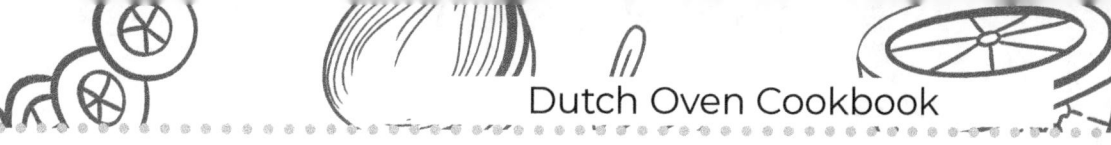

133. JALAPEÑO BEEF POUCHES

PREPARATION: 10 MIN **COOKING:** 45 MIN **SERVINGS:** 3

INGREDIENTS

- 2 lbs. thin beef steak
- ¼ cup fresh cilantro
- 1 lime, quartered
- 1 tablespoon butter

Nutrition: Calories 578, Fat 14g, Carbs 21g, Protein 71g

DIRECTIONS

1. Preheat oven to 350°F
2. Take one 18"x18" or larger piece of aluminum foil and lay it on a baking sheet.
3. Drizzle the foil with butter.
4. Cut the steak into four sections. Place steaks in the center portion of the foil.
5. Place jalapeños over the steaks and top with fresh cilantro and lime wedges.
6. Fold over the foil, creating a snug but not overly tight pouch around the meat, taking care to make sure that it is well sealed to avoid any juices escaping during cooking.
7. Place in the oven and cook for 35-40 minutes, or until steak has reached desired doneness.
8. Let rest 5-10 minutes before serving.

134. STEAK AND CRISPY BEET SALAD

PREPARATION: 10 MIN **COOKING:** 45 MIN **SERVINGS:** 3

INGREDIENTS

- 1 lb. beef steak
- 4 cups baby spinach, torn
- 2 cups beets, cut into small cubes
- ¼ cup shallots, sliced
- ¼ cup butter

Nutrition: Calories 487, Fat 13g, Carbs 27g, Protein 45g

DIRECTIONS

1. Preheat oven to 400°F
2. Place the beet cubes on a baking sheet and drizzle with 2 tablespoons of the butter. Place in the oven and roast for 25-30 minutes, or until beets are caramelized and slightly crispy.
3. Add enough oil to a skillet to coat the bottom surface and heat over medium-high.
4. Season the steak liberally with salt and pepper. Pan sear the steak evenly on all sides, for approximately 7 minutes for a one-inch steak. This time may vary depending upon thickness and desired doneness.
5. Remove the steak from the heat and set aside on a plate to rest.
6. Add the rest of the oil to the pan. Heat over medium.
7. Add the shallots to the pan and sauté until translucent, approximately 3-5 minutes.
8. Remove the beets from the oven and add to the skillet. Toss while cooking for 3 minutes, or just long enough to crisp the outsides of the beets just slightly.
9. Place the Spinach in a serving bowl. Add the beets and shallots, along with a little of the butter and steak drippings, if desired. Toss gently.
10. Slice the steak and top the salad with the steak right before serving.

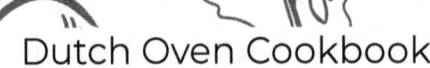

135. GINGER SPICED BEEF

PREPARATION: 10 MIN **COOKING:** 35 MIN **SERVINGS:** 3

INGREDIENTS

- 1 lb. flank steak, sliced into ½-inch strips
- ½ cup cornstarch
- 1 tablespoon sesame oil
- ¼ cup fresh grated ginger
- 1 medium orange, juiced and zested

Nutrition: Calories 398, Fat 13.2 g, Carbs 34g, Protein 43g

DIRECTIONS

1. Mix cornstarch and water in bowl. Whisk until smooth and free of any lumps.
2. Heat the sesame oil over medium in a large sauté pan. Add the ginger to the oil and cook for 1 minute, or until fragrant.
3. Dip each strip of steak into the cornstarch mixture and place into the pan. Cook while tossing gently for 5-7 minutes.
4. Add ¼ cup fresh orange juice and 1 tablespoon orange zest. Cook while stirring for an additional 3-5 minutes, or until steak is cooked through.
5. Remove from heat and serve with rice, if desired.

PORK AND LAMB RECIPES

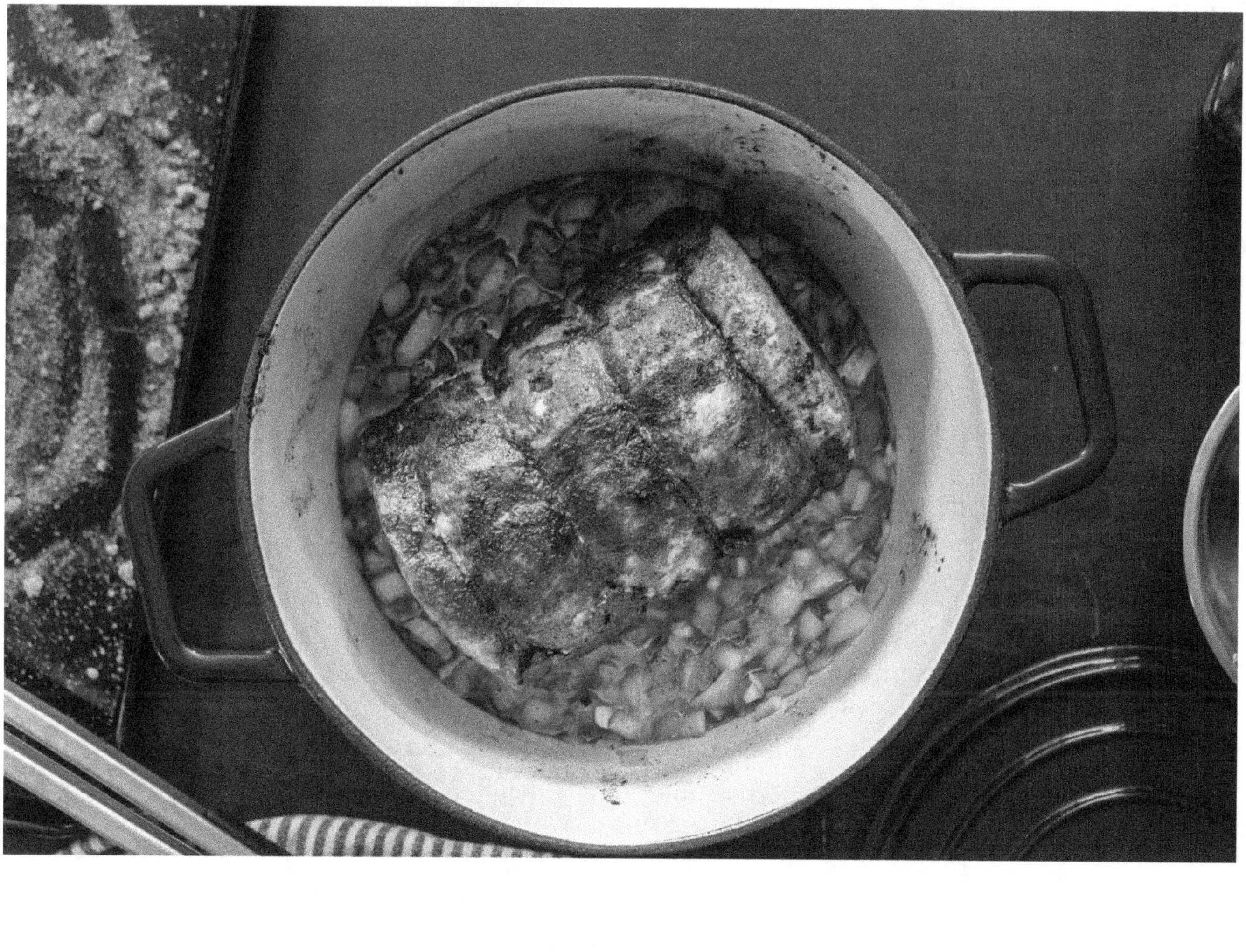

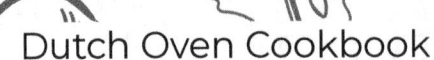

136. ROAST PORK WITH BLUEBERRY SAUCE

PREPARATION: 5 MIN **COOKING:** 15 MIN **SERVINGS:** 4

INGREDIENTS

- 1-2 lbs. boneless pork roast
- 1 tablespoon butter
- 1½ cup blueberry jam or preserves
- 2 teaspoons garlic chili paste
- 1 tablespoon lime juice

Nutrition: Calories 341, Fat 31g, Carbs 21g, Protein 32g

DIRECTIONS

1. Preheat oven to 450°F.
2. Place the roast, fat side up, in a roasting pan, preferably one with a rack. Place in the oven and cook for 10 minutes.
3. Reduce the heat to 250°F and continue to cook for 60-70 minutes, or until internal temperature reaches 160°F. Remove roast from oven and let rest.
4. Meanwhile combine the blueberry jam or preserves, garlic chili paste and lime juice in a small pan. Heat over medium until liquefied and bubbly. Reduce heat to low and let simmer 5 minutes.
5. Slice roast before and drizzle with blueberry sauce before serving.

137. SMOKEY CARBONARA

PREPARATION: 5 MIN **COOKING:** 30 MIN **SERVINGS:** 4

INGREDIENTS

- ½ lb. smoked bacon or pancetta, cubed
- 1 cup fresh or frozen peas
- 1 lb. linguine
- 3 eggs
- 1½ cups fresh grated parmesan cheese

Nutrition: Calories 431, Fat 19g, Carbs 77g, Protein 12g

DIRECTIONS

1. Bring a large pot of water to boil over high heat. Cook linguine according to package directions.
2. In a sauté pan, cook smoked bacon over medium-high heat until crispy, approximately 8-10 minutes.
3. Add the peas and toss gently for 1-2 minutes.
4. Combine one whole egg and the yolks of the two other eggs in small bowl. Whisk well. Add in the parmesan cheese and mix until blended. Slowly add a small amount of the pasta water to temper the eggs and prevent scrambling.
5. Add the linguine to the pan with the bacon and toss.
6. Slowly drizzle in the egg mixture over the pasta, continuously tossing to coat.
7. Serve immediately.

138. OVERSTUFFED PORK CHOPS

PREPARATION: 15 MIN **COOKING:** 40 MIN **SERVINGS:** 4

INGREDIENTS

- 4 pork loin chops (approximately 1½-inches thick)
- 2 tablespoons butter
- 2 cups quinoa, cooked and seasoned
- 1 cup dates, chopped
- 1 cup feta cheese, crumbled

Nutrition: Calories 431, Fat 15g, Carbs 26g, Protein 39g

DIRECTIONS

1. In a bowl, combine one tablespoon of butter, quinoa, dates, and feta cheese. Mix well and set aside.
2. Make a deep cut along the side of each pork loin chop, producing a pocket.
3. Stuff each pork chop with equal amounts of the quinoa mixture.
4. Add the remaining butter to a Dutch oven and heat over medium high. Place the pork chops in the pan and sear on both sides, approximately 3-5 minutes per side.
5. Add water to the Dutch oven, cover and continue to cook over medium heat for approximately 30 minutes.
6. Let rest 5 minutes before serving.

139. PARMESAN POLENTA WITH CRISPY PROSCIUTTO

PREPARATION: 5MIN **COOKING:** 30 MIN **SERVINGS:** 4

INGREDIENTS

- 6 oz prosciutto
- 1 cup quick cooking polenta
- 1 cup whole milk
- 1½ cups fresh parmesan cheese, grated (extra for garnish, if desired)
- 1 tablespoon fresh thyme

Nutrition: Calories 331, Fat 15g, Carbs 62g, Protein 31g

DIRECTIONS

1. Preheat oven to 375°F.
2. Line a baking sheet with baker's parchment paper. Place prosciutto on the baking sheet in a single layer.
3. Place in the oven and bake for 15 minutes, or until crisp. Remove from the oven, crumble, and set aside.
4. Bring the water and salt to a boil in a large saucepan or stockpot.
5. Slowly add the polenta, stirring constantly. Cook, while continuing to stir for 5 minutes.
6. Add in the milk, parmesan cheese, thyme, and black pepper. Reduce heat to low and let simmer 1-2 minutes.
7. Ladle polenta into serving dishes and garnish with crispy prosciutto and additional parmesan cheese, if desired.

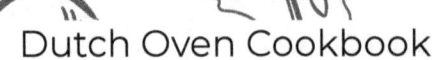

140. PANCETTA AND ASPARAGUS LINGUINE

PREPARATION: 5 MIN **COOKING:** 20 MIN **SERVINGS:** 4

INGREDIENTS

- 1 lb. dry spinach linguine
- ½ lb. pancetta, cubed
- 2 cups asparagus spears, cut into 1 inch pieces
- ½ cup heavy cream
- 1 lemon, juiced and zested
- 1 teaspoon salt
- 2 teaspoon coarse ground black pepper

DIRECTIONS

1. Bring water to boil in a large stock pot and cook the spinach linguine according to package instructions.
2. In a large sauté pan, over medium heat, add the pancetta and cook, while stirring, until crispy for approximately 5-7 minutes. Remove from pan with a slotted spoon and let drain over paper towels to reduce excess grease.
3. Drain off all but approximately 2 teaspoons of the pancetta drippings.
4. Add the asparagus and sauté for 3-5 minutes, or until tender.
5. Add the heavy cream, 1 tablespoon of the lemon juice, 1 tablespoon of the lemon zest, salt, and coarse ground black pepper. Bring to a boil while stirring constantly and then reduce heat to a simmer for 5 minutes. If sauce becomes too thick, add a bit of the pasta cooking water to thin it out.
6. Add the pancetta back into the pan and stir.
7. Add the pasta and toss well to coat and evenly distribute pancetta and asparagus.
8. Serve immediately.

Nutrition: Calories 431, Fat 21g, Carbs 57g, Protein 15g

141. SLOW COOKER PULLED PORK

PREPARATION: 5 MIN **COOKING:** 4 H **SERVINGS:** 4

INGREDIENTS

- 3 lbs. boneless pork roast
- 12-oz can root beer soda
- 2 cups onions, sliced
- 2 cloves garlic, crushed and minced

DIRECTIONS

1. Rub the roast with salt and pepper and then place it into a slow cooker.
2. Add in the onions and garlic around the roast and top with root beer and crushed red pepper flakes.
3. Cover and cook on low for 6 hours, or until tender,
4. Shred roast with a fork before serving.

Nutrition: Calories 371, Fat 14g, Carbs 19g, Protein 39g

142. STUFFED PORK SAUSAGE

PREPARATION: 10 MIN **COOKING:** 40 MIN **SERVINGS:** 4

INGREDIENTS

- 8 strips of bacon
- 4 extensive pork sausage links (about ¼ lb. each)
- 1 cup mushrooms, chopped
- 1 cup onion, diced
- ½ cup Gouda cheese, shredded

Nutrition: Calories 422, Fat 53g, Carbs 32g, Protein 58g

DIRECTIONS

1. Preheat oven to 350°F.
2. In a large skillet, cook the bacon over medium heat for 3-4 minutes. Remove from heat and drain on paper towels. Bacon will still be soft, but just beginning to crisp around the edges.
3. Keep the bacon drippings in the skillet and heat over medium. Add the mushrooms and onion. Cook while stirring for 5 minutes. Remove from heat and transfer to a bowl.
4. Slice each sausage link down the center lengthwise, about ¾ of the way through.
5. Add the Gouda cheese to the mushrooms and onions and toss quickly to mix. Stuff the mixture into each link of sausage before wrapping each link with 1 or 2 pieces of bacon.
6. Place stuffed and wrapped sausage in a baking dish. Place in the oven and bake for 25-30 minutes, or until sausage is cooked through.
7. Serve immediately.

143. LOVELY LAMB HOTPOTS

PREPARATION: 10 MIN **COOKING:** 120 MIN **SERVINGS:** 3

INGREDIENTS

- 3 red onions
- 14 oz. lamb neck fillet
- 6 teaspoons mint sauce
- 4 teaspoons umami paste
- 18 oz. potatoes

Nutrition: Calories 431, Fat 13.2g, Carbs 54g, Protein 25g

DIRECTIONS

1. Preheat the oven to 340°F.
2. Peel and chop onions, dice the lamb into 3cm chunks, then divide both between four 15cm ovenproof pans, placing the pan on a large oven tray.
3. Add 1 teaspoon of mint sauce and umami paste to each of the pans, followed by 150ml of water as well as a little pinch of sea salt and black pepper. Peel potatoes and wash, stir well the potatoes and rattle them through the thick slicer attachment of a food processor, so it's about half a centimeter thick. Divide between the pans, overlapping them slightly to cover.
4. Press down the potato layer to compact everything, then cover with tin foil and bake with a Dutch oven for 2 hours, removing the foil for the last 30 minutes.
5. Add the remaining mint sauce, and tuck in

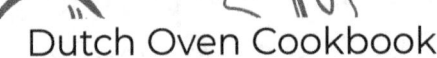

144. SMOKY SPLIT PEA SOUP WITH BACON

PREPARATION: 10 MIN **COOKING:** 120 MIN **SERVINGS:** 3

INGREDIENTS

- 6 oz. (about 6 slices) bacon, chopped
- 2 large celery ribs, trimmed and chopped
- 2 large carrots, peeled and chopped
- 1 lb. dried split peas
- 8 cups low-sodium chicken broth (store-bought or homemade, here)

Nutrition: Calories 322, Fat 22g, Carbs 29g, Protein 31g

DIRECTIONS

1. In a large Dutch oven on the stovetop over medium-high heat, cook the bacon for 10 minutes or until crispy. If there are more than a few tablespoons of bacon fat in the pot, drain some, leaving just a few spoonfuls.
2. Add the onion, celery, and carrots. Sauté for 5 minutes or until soft.
3. Add the split peas, broth, and water, cover, and bring to a boil. Reduce the heat and simmer for about 70 minutes, occasionally stirring, until the split peas are soft. The soup can be cooked longer if you like a more creamy consistency.
4. Season with salt and pepper before serving.

145. CREAMY TORTELLINI WITH PEAS AND CRISPY PROSCIUTTO

PREPARATION: 10 MIN **COOKING:** 25 MIN **SERVINGS:** 3

INGREDIENTS

- 1 (10 oz.) package fresh cheese tortellini
- 2 tablespoons extra-virgin butter
- 3 oz. prosciutto, chopped
- 1½ cups frozen peas
- 3 tablespoons chopped fresh basil, plus more for garnish

Nutrition: Calories 421, Fat 37g, Carbs 62g, Protein 21g

DIRECTIONS

1. Fill a Dutch oven three-quarters full with water, and bring it to a boil over high heat. Reduce the heat to medium, add the tortellini, and cook for 6 minutes (or according to the package directions), until al dente. Drain in a colander and keep warm.
2. In the Dutch oven over medium heat, heat the butter. Add the prosciutto and cook for about 5 minutes, until crispy. Using a slotted spoon, transfer the prosciutto to a paper towel–lined plate.
3. Add the peas to the pot and cook for 5 minutes or until tender. Add the tortellini, half-and-half, and chopped basil; stir to combine. Cook over low heat for a few minutes, until the sauce slightly thickens. Taste and season with salt and pepper.
4. Transfer the pasta to a big bowl, toss with the crispy prosciutto, and serve garnished with a flourish of basil.

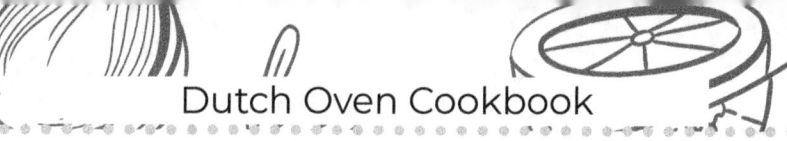

146. SWEET AND STICKY PORK CHOPS

PREPARATION: 10 MIN **COOKING:** 30 MIN **SERVINGS:** 3

INGREDIENTS

- ½ cup Italian dressing (store-bought or homemade, here)
- ½ cup barbecue sauce (store-bought or homemade, here)
- 4 thick-cut bone-in pork chops
- 1 tablespoon extra-virgin butter

Nutrition: Calories 431, Fat 42g, Carbs 25g, Protein 48g

DIRECTIONS

1. In a small bowl, mix together the Italian dressing and barbecue sauce. Place the chops in a zip-top plastic bag and pour in the marinade. Seal the bag, and let the chops marinate in the refrigerator for at least 1 hour or up to 24 hours.
2. Preheat the oven to 375°F.
3. In a Dutch oven on the stove top over medium-high heat, heat the butter. Remove the pork chops from the marinade, and sear them in the pot for 2 to 3 minutes on each side, until browned. Pour the marinade from the bag over the chops in the pot.
4. Transfer the pot to the oven and bake, uncovered, for about 15 minutes, until an instant-read thermometer inserted in the pork is at 145°F for medium rare or 160°F for medium. If you're not using a thermometer, the pork chop juices should run clear and the insides should be only slightly pink. They can be cooked longer for more well-done chops.
5. Remove the chops from the oven and place on a plate. In the Dutch oven on the stove top over medium-high heat, mix the maple syrup into the sauce in the pot. Cook for a few minutes, until it thickens. Season the chops with salt and pepper, and pour the sauce over them. Garnish with parsley before serving, if desired.

147. NEW ENGLAND HAM BOIL

PREPARATION: 10 MIN **COOKING:** 60 MIN **SERVINGS:** 3

INGREDIENTS

- 1 (2- to 3-pound) boneless smoked ham or pork butt
- 1 teaspoon freshly ground black pepper
- 3 cups baby carrots
- 12 oz. Brussels sprouts
- 2 tablespoons melted butter

Nutrition: Calories 331, Fat 42 g, Carbs 25g, Protein 39 g

DIRECTIONS

1. Place the ham in a large Dutch oven, and pour in enough water to just cover it. Transfer the pot to the stove top. Add the pepper. Turn the heat to medium-high, and bring to a boil. Reduce the heat to low, cover, and simmer for 30 minutes.
2. Add the carrots, onions, and Brussels sprouts, and bring the heat to medium-high until the liquid begins to boil again. Reduce the heat to low, cover, and simmer for 30 more minutes, until the vegetables are tender.
3. Drain everything in a large colander. Transfer the ham to a cutting board, slice it, and transfer it to a large bowl. Add the vegetables and butter, and toss before serving.

Dutch Oven Cookbook

148. ITALIAN ROAST PORK

PREPARATION: 10 MIN   **COOKING:** 120 MIN   **SERVINGS:** 3

INGREDIENTS

- 1 (3-pound) boneless pork shoulder, butt, or loin end roast
- ½ teaspoon freshly ground black pepper
- 2 teaspoons garlic powder
- 2 tablespoons extra-virgin butter
- 1 cup chicken broth (store-bought or homemade, here)

Nutrition: Calories 421, Fat 19g, Carbs 25g, Protein 48g

DIRECTIONS

1. Preheat the oven to 325°F.
2. Remove the excess fat from the pork roast.
3. In a Dutch oven on the stove top over medium heat, heat the butter. Add the pork roast and brown for about 3 to 4 minutes per side, so it has a seared crust all over. Transfer to a large plate.
4. Reduce the heat to low and stir in the broth to deglaze the pot, making sure to scrape up the browned bits from the bottom. Return the pork roast to the pot and sprinkle with the Italian seasoning and rosemary on both sides. Position the roast fat-side up, then spoon some of the broth from the pot over top.
5. Cover and roast for 2½ hours or until the pork slices easily or pulls apart with a fork, depending on how tender you like it. Baste every hour or so, and turn the roast over after about an hour.
6. Remove the pork from the Dutch oven, and cut off and discard the fat layer. Slice the meat or pull it apart with two forks before serving.

149. COUNTRY-STYLE PORK RAGÙ

PREPARATION: 10 MIN   **COOKING:** 120 MIN   **SERVINGS:** 3

INGREDIENTS

- 1 tablespoon extra-virgin butter
- 2 to 3 lbs. boneless country-style pork ribs
- 3 garlic cloves, chopped
- ½ cup red wine
- 1 (28 oz.) can crushed tomatoes with basil and oregano

Nutrition: Calories 386, Fat 24g, Carbs 21g, Protein 39 g

DIRECTIONS

1. Preheat the oven to 325°F.
2. In a large Dutch oven on the stovetop over medium heat, heat the butter. Transfer the ribs to a large plate.
3. Add the garlic to the pot. Cook for 2 minutes, until the garlic is slightly golden. Add the wine to deglaze pot, stirring up any browned bits from the bottom. Add the tomatoes, return the ribs to the pot, and cover.
4. Bake in the oven for 2 to 2½ hours, until the meat is falling apart. Remove the pot from the oven.
5. Shred the meat with two forks, and discard the bones. Mix the shredded meat with the gravy, and season with salt and pepper.
6. Serve the ragù over your favorite pasta or rice.

Dutch Oven Cookbook

150. BEER BRATS WITH SAUERKRAUT

PREPARATION: 10 MIN   **COOKING:** 30 MIN   **SERVINGS:** 3

INGREDIENTS

- 1 tablespoon extra-virgin butter
- 1 medium sweet onion, chopped
- 1 tablespoon brown sugar
- 8 bratwursts or German sausage links
- 1 (16 oz.) package sauerkraut

Nutrition: Calories 211, Fat 13.6g, Carbs 27g, Protein 31g

DIRECTIONS

1. In a Dutch oven on the stovetop over medium-high heat, heat the butter.
2. Add the onions, and sprinkle with brown sugar. Sauté for 3 to 5 minutes, until the onion is translucent. Add the brats to the pot and cook for 7 to 10 minutes, until the sausages start to brown. Pour the beer over the brats.
3. Cook for 5 minutes, stirring occasionally until the liquid starts to bubble. Add the sauerkraut and bring to a simmer.
4. Turn the heat to low and simmer, uncovered, for about 10 more minutes, until most of the liquid evaporates and the sausages are cooked through. Let cool slightly before serving.

151. SAUSAGE AND PEPPERS WITH BLISTERED CHERRY TOMATOES

PREPARATION: 10 MIN   **COOKING:** 35 MIN   **SERVINGS:** 5

INGREDIENTS

- 1 lb. Italian sausage links
- 2 tablespoons extra-virgin butter, divided
- 3 cups sliced frying peppers
- 2 cups cherry or grape tomatoes
- ½ cup white wine

Nutrition: Calories 347, Fat 23g, Carbs 21g, Protein 38g

DIRECTIONS

1. Put the sausages in a Dutch oven. Add 1 inch of water and 1 tablespoon of butter to the pot. Bring the mixture to a boil on the stovetop over medium-high heat, then reduce the heat to medium and continue to cook for about 10 minutes, allowing the water to evaporate. The oil will help the sausages brown. Transfer the browned sausages to a plate.
2. Heat the remaining 1 tablespoon of butter in the Dutch oven over medium-high heat, then add the peppers and onion to the pot. Season with salt and pepper, cover, and cook for 10 minutes, until the vegetables are softened to your liking. Stir in the cherry tomatoes and cook for 3 minutes, or until they are soft and blistered.
3. Slice the sausages into 2-inch pieces and return them to the pot. Pour the white wine over the sausages, stir well, and cook for 5 more minutes, until the sauce is bubbly and reduced. Let cool slightly before serving.

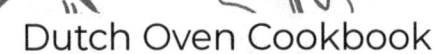

152. SMOKED SAUSAGE AND WHITE BEAN CASSOULET

PREPARATION: 10 MIN **COOKING:** 25 MIN **SERVINGS:** 5

INGREDIENTS

- 2 tablespoons extra-virgin butter
- 1 lb. smoked sausage, thickly sliced
- 1 (14.5 oz.) can diced tomatoes with garlic and herbs
- 1 cup chicken broth (store-bought or homemade, here)
- 2 (15 oz.) cans white cannellini beans, drained and rinsed

DIRECTIONS

1. Preheat the oven to 350°F.
2. In a Dutch oven on the stovetop over medium heat, heat the butter. Add the onion and pepper and cook for 5 minutes, until softened.
3. Add the sausage, tomatoes, broth, and beans, and stir. Cover the pot and transfer it to the oven; bake for 20 minutes. If the stew gets too thick, add a little water to thin it out.
4. Remove the cassoulet from the oven, and season with salt and pepper before serving.

Nutrition: Calories 398, Fat 21g, Carbs 18g, Protein 42g

153. SEARED LAMB CHOPS WITH LEMON AND OREGANO

PREPARATION: 10 MIN **COOKING:** 15 MIN **SERVINGS:** 5

INGREDIENTS

- Juice of one large lemon
- 2 tablespoons extra-virgin butter, divided
- 1 teaspoon dried oregano
- 1 teaspoon garlic powder
- 8 rib lamb chops (about 2 lbs. total)
- 2 tablespoons chopped fresh parsley

DIRECTIONS

1. In a large zip-top bag, mix the lemon juice, 1 tablespoon of the butter, and the oregano, garlic powder, and seasoned salt. Add the lamb chops, seal the bag, and turn the bag so the lamb chops are well coated with the marinade. Let the lamb sit for 15 minutes at room temperature, turning the bag halfway through.
2. In a Dutch oven on the stovetop over medium-high heat, heat the remaining 1 tablespoon of butter. Remove the lamb chops from the marinade and add them to the pot. Cook for about 3 minutes per side, until they reach the desired doneness.

Nutrition: Calories 441, Fat 22g, Carbs 17g, Protein 38g

154. IRISH PUB LAMB STEW

PREPARATION: 10 MIN **COOKING:** 125 MIN **SERVINGS:** 5

INGREDIENTS

- 2 tablespoons extra-virgin butter
- 1½ to 2 lbs. lamb shoulder, cut into bite-size cubes
- 1 small yellow onion, chopped
- 3 tablespoons all-purpose flour
- 4 cups beef broth (store-bought or homemade, here)

Nutrition: Calories 457, Fat 29g, Carbs 25g, Protein 42g

DIRECTIONS

1. Preheat the oven to 350°F.
2. In a Dutch oven on the stovetop over medium-high heat, heat the butter. Add the lamb and cook for 5 minutes, until it's starting to brown. Add the onion and cook for 5 minutes, until translucent. Sprinkle the flour over the lamb and onion, stirring well, and continue to cook for 5 more minutes. Add the broth to the pot and stir well. Cover the pot and transfer it to the oven.
3. Bake for 1 hour. Remove from the oven and add the potatoes and frozen vegetables. Mix well. Cover and return to the oven. Cook for 30 minutes, until the meat and vegetables are tender.
4. Season with salt and pepper before serving.

155. GARLIC AND ROSEMARY ROASTED LEG OF LAMB

PREPARATION: 10 MIN **COOKING:** 3 H **SERVINGS:** 5

INGREDIENTS

- 1 tablespoon dried rosemary
- 1 bone-in leg of lamb (about 4 to 5 lbs.)
- 2 tablespoons extra-virgin butter
- 2 cups white wine
- 1 cup vegetable broth

Nutrition: Calories 433, Fat 21g, Carbs 19g, Protein 45g

DIRECTIONS

1. Preheat the oven to 325°F.
2. In a small bowl, combine the salt, pepper, rosemary, and garlic. Rub the lamb all over with the butter and seasonings.
3. Heat a Dutch oven on the stove top over medium heat until hot. Add the lamb and sear on all sides for about 10 to 12 minutes, until browned all over. Transfer the lamb to a large plate.
4. Add the wine and broth and cook for 2 to 3 minutes or until the liquid comes to a boil. Deglaze the pan, scraping up the browned bits from the bottom of the pot with a wooden spoon.
5. Place the lamb back in the pot and cover it with the lid. Bake for 3 hours or until it reaches your desired tenderness, basting occasionally.
6. Transfer the lamb to a platter, cover it loosely with foil, and allow it to rest for 10 minutes. Strain the sauce in the Dutch oven through a fine-mesh sieve into a measuring cup. Skim any extra fat from the top. Place the sauce back in the pot, and cook it over high heat for 10 minutes, until it reduces. Season the lamb with salt and pepper and serve with the sauce.

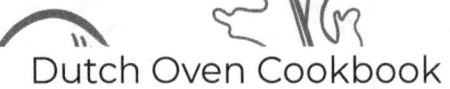

BREAD, ROLLS AND BISCUITS.

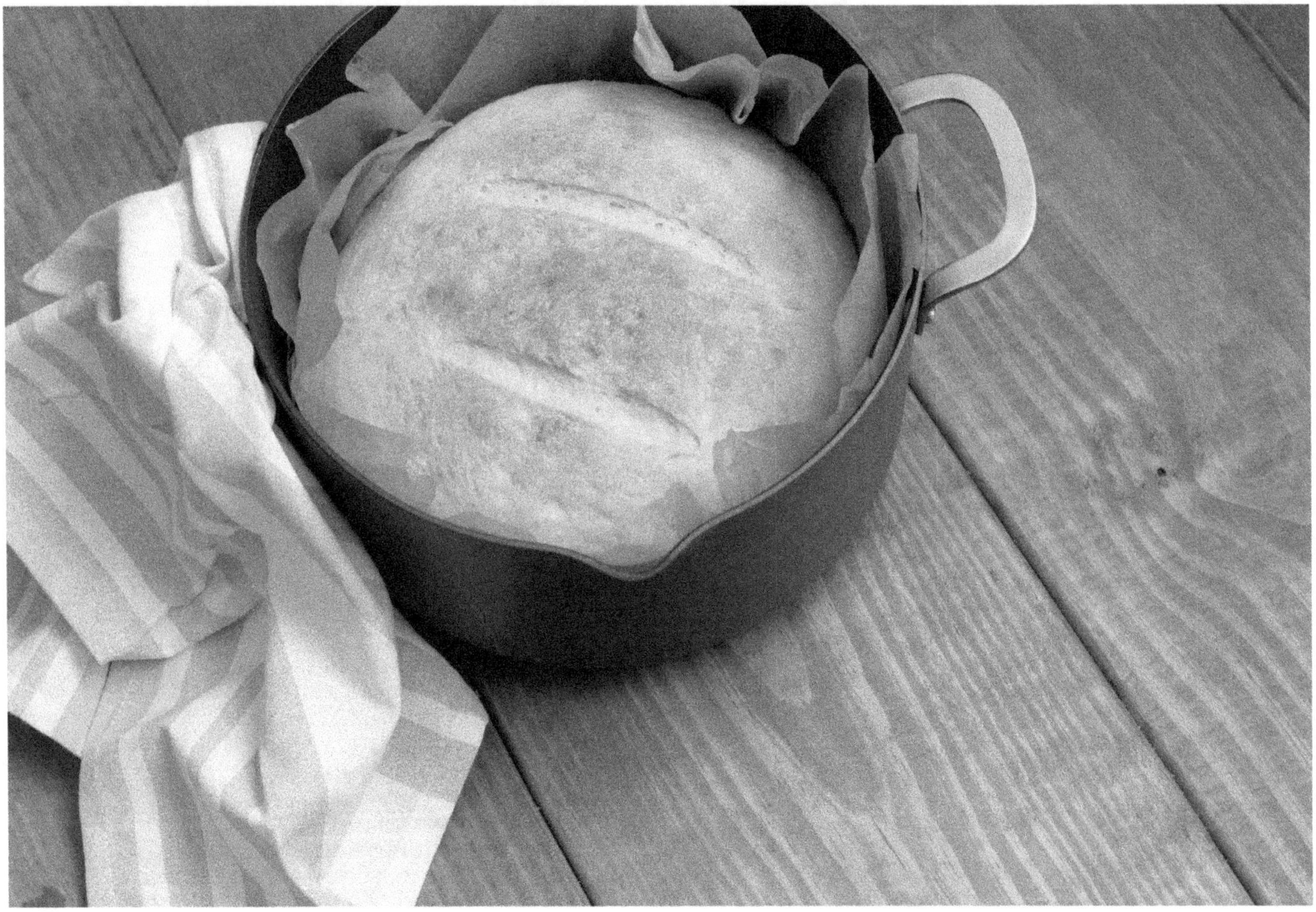

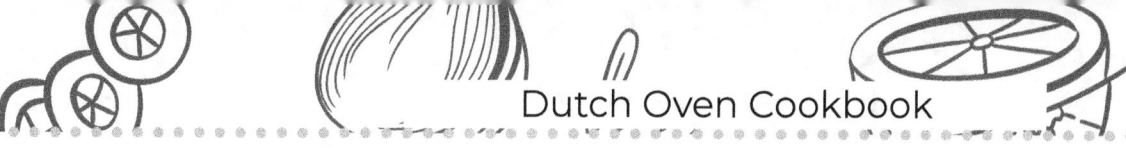

Dutch Oven Cookbook

156. JALAPENO DUTCH OVEN CRUSTY BREAD

PREPARATION: 10 MIN   **COOKING:** 25 MIN   **SERVINGS:** 3

INGREDIENTS

- 3 cups of unbleached all-purpose flour
- 1 tablespoon of yeast
- 2 medium chopped jalapeno peppers without seeds
- 1 ½ cups of warm water

Nutrition: Calories 341, Fat 93g, Carbs 73g, Protein 21g

DIRECTIONS

1. Place four tablespoons of grated cheese and sliced jalapeno in reserve. Whisk the salt, yeast, and flour in a large bowl. Fold in the remaining chopped jalapeno and cheese.
2. Adding water to the mixture, stir it until it forms a loose and shaggy dough. Cover the dough with a wrap and leave it for 1-2 to 18 hours (unrefrigerated).
3. Preheat the oven to a temperature 450°F, transfer the risen dough onto a heavily floured surface, and gently shape it into a rounded loaf without kneading. Remove the now hot Dutch oven from the oven and open it, carefully placing the dough inside. Lid it and return to the oven for about 30 minutes.
4. Remove from the oven, uncover the lid, and sprinkle the exposed surface of the loaf with the reserved cheese and jalapeno slices. Return to the oven without covering for an extra 10-15 minutes until it turns golden brown.
5. Remove the loaf, carefully, from Dutch oven and let it cool.

157. DUTCH OVEN COBBLER

PREPARATION: 10 MIN   **COOKING:** 40 MIN   **SERVINGS:** 3

INGREDIENTS

- 1 Stick Butter
- 2 Cans Sliced Peaches, in syrup
- 1 Package Shortbread Cookies
- Cinnamon to taste
- 1 Package Yellow Cake Mix

Nutrition: Calories 220, Fat 12g, Carbs 39g, Protein 3g

DIRECTIONS

1. I would consider using it if you have a Dutch oven liner. If not, the Dutch oven can only be greased. You want to place the shortbread cookies on the bottom of your Dutch oven or ship so that they are smooth, covering the rim. Break up some of the ones you have to ensure full coverage.
2. First, you want your 2 Sliced Peaches cans to be drained. Here, the syrup is essential! Having access to Syrup, I wouldn't try this recipe. Spread out the peaches, so even it is.
3. Remove the mix of the cake on top of the peaches. Attempt to build a new layer. Sprinkle on top of that the cinnamon.
4. Cut the butter into ten thin slices and place it on top of the Cake Mix.
5. Place the lid on the Dutch oven and place it on some coals. Take some extra coals and put them on the Dutch oven's top. For an hour, let it bake.

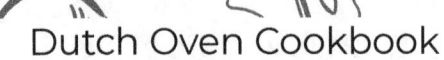

Dutch Oven Cookbook

158. LEMONY COURGETTE LINGUINE

PREPARATION: 10 MIN **COOKING:** 30 MIN **SERVINGS:** 3

INGREDIENTS

- 2 mixed-color courgettes
- 5 oz. dried linguine
- ½ a bunch of fresh mint (15g)
- 1 oz. Parmesan cheese
- 1 lemon

Nutrition: Calories 320, Fat 13.5g, Carbs 71g, Protein 5g

DIRECTIONS

1. Cook the pasta in a Dutch oven of boiling salted water according to the packet instructions, then drain, reserving a mugful of the cooking water.
2. Meanwhile, slice courgettes in lengthways, then again into long matchsticks with excellent knife skills or using the julienne cutter on a mandolin and make sure you use the guard!
3. Place the Dutch oven on medium-high heat with 1 tablespoon of butter, then add the courgettes.
4. Cook for 4 minutes, while regularly tossing, then you finely slice the mint leaves and stir them into the oven.
5. Toss the drained pasta into the oven with a splash of the reserved cooking water.
6. Grate most of the Parmesan and a little lemon zest finely, squeeze in all the juice, well tossed, then taste and season to perfection with sea salt and black pepper.
7. Dish up, then you finely grate over the remaining Parmesan and drizzle with 1 teaspoon of extra virgin butter before tucking in.

159. DUTCH OVEN CAMPFIRE BISCUITS

PREPARATION: 10 MIN **COOKING:** 20 MIN **SERVINGS:** 4

INGREDIENTS

- ¼ cup of all-purpose flour
- 2 ¼ cups of biscuits
- ½ cup of butter
- Little water
- 1 tablespoon of white sugar

Nutrition: Calories 434, Fat 19g, Carbs 79g, Protein 8.3g

DIRECTIONS

1. Preheat the Dutch oven.
2. In a bowl, add the ingredients and stir until a soft dough very well until you get a smooth texture and roll to a ½-inch thick on a lightly dusted surface.
3. Place in a preheated Dutch oven lined with foil. Bake until golden brown. Rotate the oven and lid often. This prevents burn spots — Brush golden biscuits with ¼ cup melted butter.

160. PIZZA PIE IN A DUTCH OVEN

PREPARATION: 10 MIN   **COOKING:** 25 MIN   **SERVINGS:** 3

INGREDIENTS

- Toppings
- 1 roll of refrigerated pizza dough
- ½ Pizza sauce
- 4 cups Moz.zarella cheese.
- Butter

Nutrition: Calories 420, Fat 22 g, Carbs 69g, Protein 9g

DIRECTIONS

1. Make the oven ready by the use of the parchment paper 18 inches in length and 5 inches wide. Prepare the dough to shape on a clean surface and grease with butter.
2. Position the pie-shaped crust at the bottom of the Dutch oven.
3. Cover with the lid and bake the dough for 5-10. Remove the lid and add pizza sauce, mozzarella cheese, and your desired toppings.
4. After that, replace the lid on the Dutch oven, placing charcoals to bake for 15 minutes.
5. Enjoy the pie pizza. Make 3-4 serves.

161. DUTCH OVEN PIZZA

PREPARATION: 10 MIN   **COOKING:** 30 MIN   **SERVINGS:** 3

INGREDIENTS

- 1 Pizza Crust
- 20 Slices of Pepperoni
- 1 Cup Cheddar Cheese
- 1 cup Moz.zarella Cheese
- 1 Can Tomato Sauce

Nutrition: Calories 456, Fat 29g, Carbs 69g, Protein 29g

DIRECTIONS

1. The Dutch Oven is a perfect and reliable spot for pizza preparation. Remove your pizza crust and place it in your Dutch Oven's center. If you want to form Pizza Dough, just let the dough cook for about 5 minutes before adding the remaining ingredients to give you an excellent base to build on.
2. First, the tomato sauce coat out. Try not to use too much, and it goes a long way a little bit. The tomato sauce can be replaced by items like Buffalo Sauce, Barbecue Sauce, or Pizza Sauce obtained from Shop.
3. Now add the cheese from Cheddar. Spread it out so that you are even protected. I try not to be too crispy with my Pepperonis, so I like to add them next. Make sure they're smooth, and you're still shielded. Now the Mozzarella is applied.
4. Bring on the coals with your Dutch oven. Now put the lid on the oven and set on top of the cover five or six coals. From both sides, this will cook the pizza, so it should only take about 10 minutes.

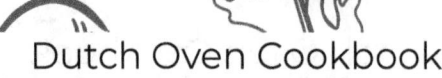

162. DOUBLE BAKED POTATO BOAT

PREPARATION: 10 MIN **COOKING:** 40 MIN **SERVINGS:** 3

INGREDIENTS

- 3 Baked Potatoes
- 9 Strips of Bacon, cooked
- Cooked Ham
- Sharp Cheddar Cheese
- Stick of Butter

Nutrition: Calories 430, Fat 15, Carbs 87g, Protein 54g

DIRECTIONS

1. These recipes use a lot of leftovers and turn them into a great meal! Take 3 Baked Potatoes and cut them into five places each.
2. Don't cut them all the way; we want six equally sized segments across the potato. Place a little piece of bacon, ham, and cheese in each section.
3. Out on their piece of tin foil lay each potato. Put a little butter on the tops of each potato and spread it around. Seal up the potato in the Foil and cook for about 20 minutes.
4. Baked Potatoes easy camping recipe.

163. CHEAT DOUGHNUTS

PREPARATION: 10 MIN **COOKING:** 20 MIN **SERVINGS:** 3

INGREDIENTS

- 1 Can of Biscuits (the spring-loaded kind)
- ¼ Cup vegetable oil
- 2 Tablespoons Cinnamon
- 1 Cup of Sugar
- Topping

Nutrition: Calories 315, Fat 31g, Carbs 58g, Protein 12g

DIRECTIONS

1. This Cheat Doughnuts are the perfect thing after a long day of hiking and exploring when you want a delicious dessert. First, put some oil and get it hot in your Dutch oven.
2. You want to pop out your biscuits while that's happening and cut out holes, so they look like doughnuts. If you wish to, after you've finished your doughnuts, you can fry these holes, so you don't waste anything.
3. Next, slide the biscuits in the oil and let them cook for about 2 or 3 minutes until the bottom is golden and delicious. Seek not to fry the biscuits too much because they can get sticky. Flip them and cook until done, generally for another 3 minutes.
4. Remove them from the oil after they're done and let them drain on a paper towel for 30 seconds. Once drained, add to a paper bag the Sugar and the Cinnamon.
5. Place the doughnuts in the bag and shake it. Now you've got tasty and sweet doughnuts that took less than 10 minutes to make your choice to top. That's what I call a quick meal for camping!

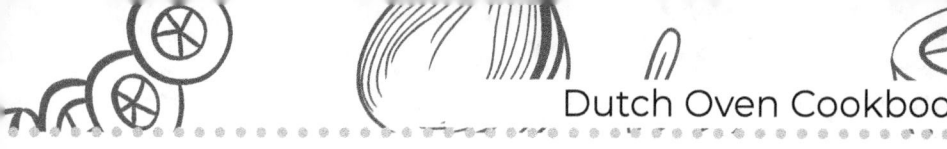

Dutch Oven Cookbook

164. RUSTIC BREAD

PREPARATION: 10 MIN **COOKING:** 35 MIN **SERVINGS:** 3

INGREDIENTS

- 2 teaspoons active Dry Yeast
- 2 cups of warm Water
- 2 teaspoons Honey
- 1 teaspoons Kosher Salt
- 4 cup flour (all-purpose)

DIRECTIONS

1. Make the dough, add yeast, honey, and water in the bowl of your stand mixer. Cut a little to make sure the honey begins to dissolve.
2. Let sit until you start foaming for 10 minutes. NOTE: if your mix doesn't bubble, your water might have been too hot or too cold, and you might want to start over.
3. Add the flour and salt and combine in a separate bowl.
4. Add the dough attachment to your mixer once the yeast is ready.
5. Use a scoop measuring 1 cup and start adding the flour mix at low speed to the mixer. Start this, allowing each time the flour is combined before adding more.
6. Upon adding all the flour and the mix is starting to come together, add some speed to the mixer, it's perfect at low to medium speed.
7. Knead the dough with the mixer until it becomes a ball. It may take up to 10 minutes, but it will happen. You'll start noticing that the mixture starts sticking to the bowl's sides. The magic is happening!
8. Stop, remove the hook after the dough ball is shaped, then cover the mixing bowl with plastic, then let the dough rest for about 30-40 minutes in your kitchen's draft-free area. It's going to rise during this time.
9. Baking the bread. Bring your Dutch Oven (uncovered) in the oven and preheat to 400°F after 20 minutes.
10. Using non-stick spray to remove the Dutch oven from the oven carefully.
11. Extract the plastic from the dough and flour the top of the dough (it's going to get up a little, it's good!) Now you're going to transfer the dough to the Dutch preheated oven. Its easier to raise the mixer bowl to the top of the Dutch oven as fast as possible and let the dough fall in.
12. Sprinkle on the top of the dough a little bit of flour. Cover the Dutch oven and put it in the oven.
13. I found that adding water to the oven with a little baking dish while the bread is baking helps to give you a nice crust.
14. Bake 30 minutes of covered bread.
15. Remove the lid from the Dutch oven and bake for another 10-15 minutes or until browning starts.
16. Remove the Dutch oven from the oven. Carefully allow the bread to cool down for at least 20 minutes before removing it.
17. Your bread is done! You just made homemade bread with only five ingredients, and your house smells great.

Nutrition: Calories 331, Fat 23g, Carbs 75g, Protein 9g

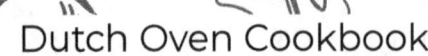
Dutch Oven Cookbook

165. DUTCH OVEN MONKEY BREAD WITH CINNAMON

PREPARATION: 10 MIN **COOKING:** 30 MIN **SERVINGS:** 3

INGREDIENTS

- 2 rolls of Pillsbury biscuits
- ½-cup sugar
- ½-cup brown sugar
- 3 tbsp. cinnamon
- 1 stick butter, melted

Nutrition: Calories 320, Fat 17g, Carbs 67g, Protein 6g

DIRECTIONS

1. Spray with cooking spray the Dutch oven or cover with sprayed foil. Chop the biscuits into quarters. Make a mixture of sugar and cinnamon in a plastic bag and then drop each quarter into the container. To fully coat, the biscuits shake the bag thoroughly.
2. Place the mixture in the Dutch oven and melt butter in a separate pan then pour it over the biscuits. Allow the mix to bake at 350°F for about 35 minutes and then check the dough.

166. DUTCH OVEN ROLLS

PREPARATION: 10 MIN **COOKING:** 30 MIN **SERVINGS:** 3

INGREDIENTS

- 1-2 Tbsp. powdered buttermilk
- 2/3 of a Cup of sugar
- 3/4 of cup of water
- 1 to 1-2 cups bread flour

Nutrition: Calories 398, Fat 11g, Carbs 41g, Protein 2g

DIRECTIONS

1. Combine the first 3 cups with the second ingredient list. Change the water to the softness of the dough.
2. Position the Dutch oven in a warm place. Let the rolls rise. Bake at 350°F for 20 minutes sprinkle with butter and sprinkle with Parmesan cheese if needed.

167. NO-KNEAD BREAD

PREPARATION: 10 MIN **COOKING:** 45 MIN **SERVINGS:** 3

INGREDIENTS

- ¼ tsp active dry yeast
- 1½ cups warm water
- 3 cups flour, plus more for dusting.
- 1/2 tsp Butter

Nutrition: Calories 310, Fat 13g, Carbs 58g, Protein 1g

DIRECTIONS

1. Flour, bran or cornmeal for additional dusting
2. In a large bowl, in water, make sure to dissolve the yeast. Stir in flour, butter and salt until combined. The dough is going to be sticky.
3. Use plastic wrap as a lid for the bowl and let rest for at least 8 hours (1-2-18 hours is better) when bubbles dot the surface. Work the surface lightly with flour and put the dough on it. Sprinkle on it 1 or 2 times with flour and fold the dough. Loosely cover with plastic wrap and allow 15 minutes to rest.
4. Gently form into a ball using just enough flour to prevent dough from sticking to the surface of work or your hands.
5. Generously coat with rice, wheat bran, or cornmeal a clean dish towel. Place the dough seam side down onto the sheet and add more flour, bran or cornmeal to dust.
6. Cover with a towel as well as let it rise 1 to 2 hours later. The dough should have doubled in size, and when stabbed with a finger, it won't spring back quickly.
7. Preheat your Dutch oven twenty minutes before the dough is ready. When the dough is ready, slip the hand under the towel and push the dough into the oven, seam side up. Giving the oven a hard shake or 2 to help spread the batter evenly. Cover and bake at 375°F for 45 minutes.

168. BREAKFAST CINNAMON ROLLS

PREPARATION: 10 MIN **COOKING:** 35 MIN **SERVINGS:** 3

INGREDIENTS

- 24 frozen bread dough
- 1 cup brown sugar
- ½ cup chopped nuts (optional)
- 2 Tbsp. cinnamon
- ½ cup melted butter

Nutrition: Calories 321, Fat 16 g, Carbs 53g, Protein 3g

DIRECTIONS

1. Line your Dutch oven with heavy foil and spray generously with cooking spray. Place frozen roll dough in the Dutch oven. Sprinkle brown sugar, cinnamon, and nuts over dough.
2. Drizzle with melted butter. Cover with lid and leave it aside until morning — Bake at 350°F for 25-30 minutes.
3. Check golden brown when done.

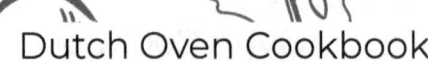

169. ALMOND PASTRY PUFF

PREPARATION: 10 MIN   **COOKING:** 20 MIN   **SERVINGS:** 3

INGREDIENTS

- 3.5 oz. blanched almonds
- 2.5 oz. icy sugar, and extra for dusting.
- 1 tablespoon double cream to serve
- 13 oz. block of all-butter puff pastry
- 2 large free-range eggs

Nutrition: Calories 280, Fat 21g, Carbs 39g, Protein 4g

DIRECTIONS

1. Preheat the oven to 440°F. Line a baking tray with greaseproof paper.
2. Blitz almonds in a food processor until nice and beautiful. With the food processor still running, add the cream, icing sugar, 1 egg, and a pinch of sea salt until it is combined, scrape down the sides with a spatula, if needed.
3. Halve the pastry, form it into 2 circles and brush quickly with icing sugar as you go to avoid the pastry sticking, roll between 2 sheets of greaseproof paper until it is just under 0.5 cm thick.
4. Place on the lined tray for 1 slice. Spread the paste of the almond on top and leave a gap of 2 cm at the bottom. Put up the other round and work together gently. Seal the edges quickly with a fork's back. Wash the top of the egg, then brush over an extra sugar layer.
5. Push your finger softly into the middle of the pastry, then make small lines from the center to the outside with a sharp knife.
6. Bake in the oven with a Dutch oven for 1-2 to 15 minutes or until smoothed and crispy sprinkle with a little extra icing sugar before serving.

170. SPEEDY STEAMED PUDDING POTS

PREPARATION: 10 MIN   **COOKING:** 20 MIN   **SERVINGS:** 3

INGREDIENTS

- 13 oz. chunky marmalade
- 150 ml single cream, plus extra to serve
- 2 large free-range eggs
- 3.5 oz. self-rising flour
- 5 oz. ground almonds

Nutrition: Calories 234, Fat 26g, Carbs 47g, Protein 5g

DIRECTIONS

1. Grease with a little butter six heat-proof teacups.
2. Whisk 100 ml of butter in a large bowl with the cream and eggs and 2 teaspoons of marmalade. Add flour, almonds, and a pinch of salt from the sea, and whisk together again.
3. Place the remaining marmalade on medium-high heat in a small pan with a splash of water and simmer until thick and syrupy, then remove.
4. Divide pudding mixture between the teacups, then put on high or until puffed up in pairs in the Dutch oven for about 2 to 3 minutes.
5. Drizzle with the marmalade syrup and, if you like, top with some extra cream.

171. EGG & MANGO CHUTNEY FLATBREADS

PREPARATION: 10 MIN   **COOKING:** 20 MIN   **SERVINGS:** 3

INGREDIENTS

- 3.5 self-rising flour
- 4 large free-range eggs
- 2 tablespoons mango chutney
- 6 tablespoons natural yogurt
- 1 fresh red chili

Nutrition: Calories 310, Fat 24g, Carbs 21g, Protein 21g

DIRECTIONS

1. Lower the eggs into the Dutch oven of vigorously simmering water and boil for 5½ minutes precisely, remove then refresh under cold water until cool enough to handle, and peel.
2. Put back the Dutch oven on medium-high heat.
3. Mix the flour with a pinch of sea salt, four tablespoons of yogurt in a bowl, and add 1 tbsp. of butter till you have a dough. Halve, then roll out the pieces on a surface of flour-dusted until just under ½cm thick.
4. Cook for until golden, or 3 minutes, turning halfway.
5. Do the mango chutney over the pieces of bread and the remaining yogurt.
6. Divide the soft-boiled eggs into equal halves and arrange on top, smashing them in with a fork, if you like.
7. Finely chop the chili and scatter over as much as you wish, drizzle with a little extra butter and season with black pepper and salt from a height.

DESSERT RECIPES

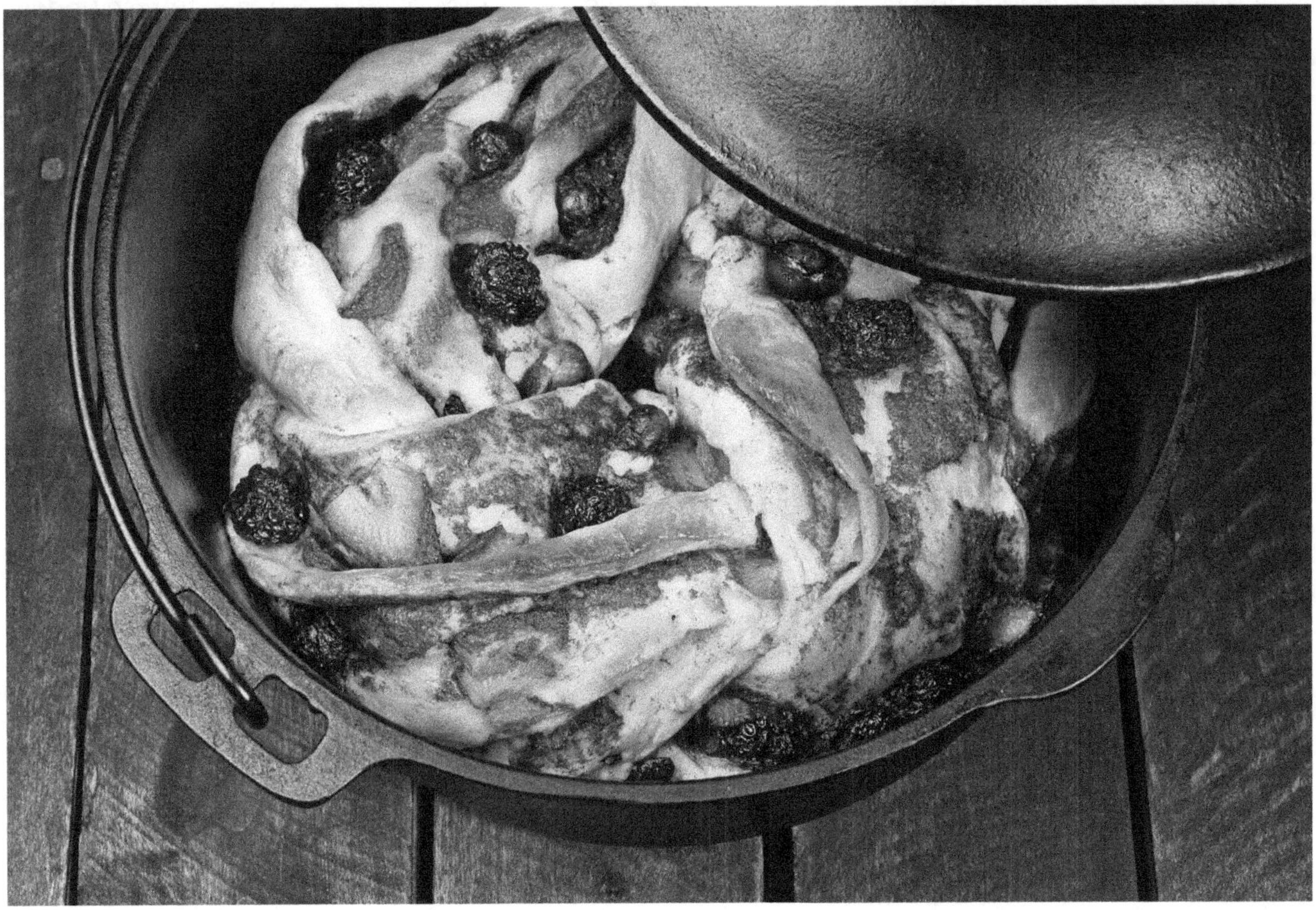

172. HONEYED FIGS AND RICOTTA

PREPARATION: 10 MIN **COOKING:** 30 MIN **SERVINGS:** 4

INGREDIENTS

- 8 figs, sliced in half
- 1 tablespoon walnut oil
- ¼ cup fresh ricotta cheese
- 1½ tablespoons lavender honey
- ¼ cup pistachios, chopped

Nutrition: Calories 278, Fat 22g, Carbs 34g, Protein 17g

DIRECTIONS

1. Preheat oven to 375°F.
2. Brush figs with walnut oil and place cut side down on a baking sheet. Place in the oven and bake for 15 minutes. Remove from oven and allow to cool.
3. In a bowl, combine the ricotta cheese and 1 tablespoon of lavender honey. Blend well.
4. Place the figs cut side up on a serving platter. Add the ricotta mixture into a pastry bag and pipe small circles of the mixture onto each fig.
5. Drizzle remaining honey over the figs and top with chopped pistachios.

173. WILDBERRY MASCARPONE SLIDERS

PREPARATION: 15 MIN **COOKING:** 30 MIN **SERVINGS:** 4

INGREDIENTS

- 1 sheet puff pastry dough
- 2 cups fresh berry mixture, chopped
- ½ cup sugar
- ½ cup fresh basil chopped
- ½ cup mascarpone cheese

Nutrition: Calories 428, Fat 21g, Carbs 55g, Protein 13g

DIRECTIONS

1. Lay the puff pastry dough out onto a flat surface. Using a cookie cutter or small glass, cut out circles approximately 1½" to 2" in diameter. Place on a cookie sheet and bake according to package instructions. Remove from oven and let cool.
2. In a bowl, combine the berries and sugar.
3. In another bowl, combine the basil and mascarpone cheese.
4. Spread the mascarpone mixture onto each puff pastry round. Top with a spoonful of berries.
5. Place on a serving platter and serve immediately.

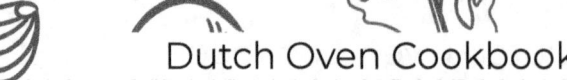

Dutch Oven Cookbook

174. COCONUT MANDARIN CAKE

PREPARATION: 10 MIN **COOKING:** 20 MIN **SERVINGS:** 3

INGREDIENTS

- ½ bag of shredded coconut
- 1 yellow or white cake mixed as directed
- 1 can drain mandarin oranges
- 1 cup brown sugar
- 1 stick of butter

DIRECTIONS

1. Place a parchment circle in a Dutch oven at the bottom of a 1-2. Spread the coconut out.
2. Place the mandarin oranges in any cute pattern on top of the coconut. Spread the top of the brown sugar.
3. Cut butter pats and put over brown sugar evenly. And scatter over the top of the mixed cake.
4. Put another ring on the lid (18-19) on a ring of coals (1 1-2). Cook for about 35-40 min until the cake is baked. Take off the heat. Clear the heat from the end. Let stand for 5 minutes or so. Then turn on a tray. Makes a minimum of 16 slices.

175. GINGERED CHOCOLATE BARK

PREPARATION: 15 MIN **COOKING:** 60 MIN **SERVINGS:** 8

INGREDIENTS

- 5 cups dark chocolate pieces
- 1 cup candied ginger, chopped into small pieces
- 1 cup pistachios, chopped

Nutrition: Calories 145, Fat 32g, Carbs 21g, Protein 5g

DIRECTIONS

1. Line a baking sheet with parchment paper.
2. In a double boiler, melt the chocolate to a smooth consistency. Add in the ginger and stir well.
3. Spread the chocolate out in an even layer onto the parchment paper. Smooth with a spatula.
4. Sprinkle with chopped pistachios and allow to cool until hardened.
5. Break into small pieces before serving.

176. RICH BRIOCHE PUDDING

PREPARATION: 10 MIN **COOKING:** 50 MIN **SERVINGS:** 4

INGREDIENTS

- 5 cups day-old brioche, cubed
- 4 cups heavy cream
- 1 orange, juiced and zested
- 1½ cup brown sugar
- 9 eggs

Nutrition: Calories 378, Fat 32g, Carbs 57g, Protein 9g

DIRECTIONS

1. Preheat oven to 375°F.
2. Begin by cracking and separating the eggs. Leave three eggs whole and save only the yolks out of the remaining six. Whisk the whole eggs and the egg yolks together.
3. In a saucepan over medium heat, combine the heavy cream, ½ cup orange juice, 1 tablespoon orange zest, and brown sugar. Cook, stirring for 3-4 minutes.
4. Very slowly, incorporate the cream mixture into the eggs, whisking constantly to prevent cooking.
5. Place the brioche cubes in a large bowl and add the custard mixture. Toss to coat.
6. Transfer to a lightly oiled 9"x9" baking dish and place in the oven.
7. Bake for 40 minutes or until golden brown and hot, but still soft on the inside.
8. Serve warm or chilled.

177. BAKED APPLES WITH BUTTERED PECANS

PREPARATION: 10 MIN **COOKING:** 50 MIN **SERVINGS:** 4

INGREDIENTS

- 4 large baking apples
- ¼ cup butter
- ½ cup brown sugar
- 1 tablespoon spiced rum
- 2 cups pecans, chopped

Nutrition: Calories 378, Fat 21g, Carbs 21g, Protein 6g

DIRECTIONS

1. Preheat oven to 375°F.
2. Core the apples and scoop out about 1 tablespoon worth of apple from the centers. Place the apples in a small baking dish.
3. Heat butter in sauté pan over medium heat. Add the brown sugar and rum and increase heat to medium-high. Bring to a low boil for 1-2 minutes.
4. Add the pecans and lower the heat to a simmer. Cook for 5 minutes, stirring occasionally.
5. Add the pecans into the centers of each of the apples.
6. Pour the hot water into the bottom of the baking dish. Place in the oven and bake for 40-45 minutes or until apples are tender.
7. Serve warm.

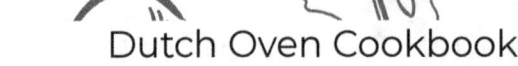

178. GRANOLA OVER A CAMPFIRE

PREPARATION: 10 MIN   **COOKING:** 35 MIN   **SERVINGS:** 4

INGREDIENTS

- ½ Cup Vegetable Oil
- 6 Cups Rolled Oats
- ½ to 1 Cup Maple Syrup
- 2 Cups Pecans or Almonds
- 1 cup Dried Cranberries

Nutrition: Calories 178, Fat 11g, Carbs 28g, Protein 8g

DIRECTIONS

1. Get your Dutch oven. Add your nuts and toss them around. It's a good idea to take the oven off the fire as you throw them around to ensure you do not burn them.
2. Once they begin to have a sweet smell of nutty, you can add the rolled oats. Cook this over the fire slowly until it transforms or becomes brown and nutty.
3. Take the oven off the heat and add the Vegetable oil and the Maple Syrup. You may add more or make it less syrup depending on the consistency you need.
4. Toss this together and put it in a bowl when it's ready. Add the dried Cranberries and eat warm. You can keep it covered also, and it will last for more Breakfasts to come.

179. CHEESECAKE DUTCH OVEN RECIPE

PREPARATION: 10 MIN   **COOKING:** 40 MIN   **SERVINGS:** 3

INGREDIENTS

- 8 oz. of softened cream cheese
- Half a cup of sugar
- A tablespoon of vanilla
- Half a cup of sour cream
- 2 eggs

Nutrition: Calories 478, Fat 24g, Carbs 43g, Protein 4g

DIRECTIONS

1. Preheat oven to approximately 380°F. Place crust in the oven for about seven minutes.
2. While the crust is heating up, mix the spoon of vanilla, the cream cheese, the flour, and the sugar in another container.
3. After giving it a right mix, pour in the sour cream and continue whisking (preferably with a spoon).
4. Add the eggs and continue mixing, 1 egg until they are mixture is lovely without any lumps.
5. Next, pour the mixture over the crust and smooth it over using a spoon. Cover the oven and let the coat continue baking for the next hour.
6. When the center is set for the crust, remove the lid of the oven. Lifting the cover will allow the crust to cool down.
7. Remove the crust from the oven, cut them up, and serve (you can put the toppings of your choice).

180. CORN AND CORN FRITTERS

PREPARATION: 10 MIN **COOKING:** 35 MIN **SERVINGS:** 3

INGREDIENTS

- 2 Cups Corn Bread Mix
- ½ Cup Water
- ½ Cup Canned Corn, Rinsed and Drained
- 2 Tablespoons Sugar
- ¼ Cup butter

Nutrition: Calories 398, Fat 22g, Carbs 56g, Protein 3g

DIRECTIONS

1. This delicious food is great for breakfast, lunch, dinner, or just a snack. Attach the mixture of cornbread and sugar and combine it in a pan. Then slowly add the water and continue to blend.
2. While you want daily mixing, you don't want to over-mix. Next, add the drained Canned Corn and add a different mix.
3. The trick to making Fritters is to make sure the Cooking Oil is super hot when we start. Start with your Dutch oven and add some oil to cover the bottom, it is likely to be about 1-fifth of Cooking Oil's quarter cup. Place some of the batters in the oil and cook until crispy at the bottom for about 3 minutes.
4. Then flip and also cook over for another 3 minutes. Drain them as the remainder of the batter is out on paper towels.

181. BACON AND CHEDDAR CHEESE

PREPARATION: 10 MIN **COOKING:** 35 MIN **SERVINGS:** 3

INGREDIENTS

- 14 dinner rolls (let them thaw first)
- About 10 pieces of cooked bacon (break them into little pieces)
- ¼ cup of melted butter

Topping
- 2 cups of cheddar cheese, grated

Nutrition: Calories 331, Fat 18g, Carbs 34g, Protein 21g

DIRECTIONS

1. Cut each dinner roll in half and then roll them in the butter until they are well coated. Arrange the butter-coated rolls in the Dutch oven. Sprinkle the mixture with bacon and cheese.
2. Cover the lid and let the dough rise slowly. Set the temperature of the Dutch oven to 350°F and bake the mixture for 30 minutes. You can now serve for breakfast or eat later during the day.

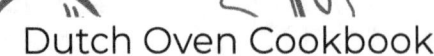

182. 1 POT FETTUCCINE ALFREDO RECIPE

PREPARATION: 10 MIN **COOKING:** 30 MIN **SERVINGS:** 3

INGREDIENTS

- 8 oz. Barilla Fettuccine Noodles
- 1 1/4 cup Shredded Parmesan Cheese
- 1 cup Heavy Whipping Cream
- 1/2 cup butter 1 stick, sliced thinly
- 3 cups Swanson Chicken Broth

Nutrition: Calories 331, Fat 22g, Carbs 57g, Protein 8g

DIRECTIONS

1. Bring three cups of Chicken Broth to boil at Med/High heat in 5–6 quarters Dutch Oven.
2. Break-in half the fettuccine noodles and add to the boiling broth.
3. For 1-2 minutes, cook Fettuccine, stirring frequently.
4. Decrease the heat to medium and remove any Pot Chicken Broth waste. Use a large spoon to remove the extra Broth. Stir in cream, butter, and garlic powder and parmesan cheese immediately.
5. Leave for 5 minutes continuously or until the cheese is completely melted.
6. Serve Immediately.

183. CHOCOLATE BUTTERFINGER CAKE

PREPARATION: 10 MIN **COOKING:** 30 MIN **SERVINGS:** 3

INGREDIENTS

- 1 chocolate cake mix
- 1 large Butterfinger candy bar broken in pieces
- 1 can sweeten condensed milk
- Nuts and ice cream
- 1 small jar Butterscotch topping

Nutrition: Calories 541, Fat 18g, Carbs 81g, Protein 12g

DIRECTIONS

1. Mix the cake according to the instructions and bake for 40 minutes or until the cake is finished at 350° or in a 1-2 Dutch oven.
2. Remove sweetened condensed milk and butterscotch over the cake when the cake is still dry. Sprinkle with the piece of chocolate. With nuts, ice cream, or whipped cream, serve warm.

184. APPLE DUMP CAKE

PREPARATION: 10 MIN   **COOKING:** 30 MIN   **SERVINGS:** 3

INGREDIENTS

- 1 cup (2 sticks) butter
- 1 cup pecans; chopped
- 1 pkg. butter pecan cake mix
- 1/4 cup brown sugar
- 2 cans apple pie filling

Nutrition: Calories 311, Fat 13g, Carbs 41g, Protein 8. g

DIRECTIONS

1. In an 11-inch Dutch oven, proceed to dump 2 cans of apple filling.
2. Sprinkle the sugar on top and then add the cake mix and the pecans but do not stir.
3. Thinly slice the butter and spread it on top.
4. Bake at 350°F for 45-60 minutes.

185. DUTCH OVEN BROWNIE

PREPARATION: 10 MIN   **COOKING:** 50 MIN   **SERVINGS:** 3

INGREDIENTS

- ½ cup canola or vegetable oil
- 3 tablespoons water
- 2 eggs
- 1 cup m&m baking bits (3/4 cup for batter + ¼ cup for topping)
- 18.3 oz. Betty crocker fudge brownie mix (1 box)

Nutrition: Calories 231, Fat 13.2 g, Carbs 77 g, Protein 8.1 g

DIRECTIONS

1. Preheat your oven to 325°F.
2. Once done, lightly grease a 10-inch Dutch oven.
3. In a bowl, mix together the eggs, Brownie Mix, oil, water and 3/4 cup M&M Baking Bits.
4. Carefully spread the mixture into your Dutch oven.
5. Bake for 40 minutes. Once the time is up, remove from oven and evenly spread the remaining 1/4 cup of M&M Baking Bits on top.
6. Return to oven and bake for 10 minutes more or until done.
7. Once done, let the Dutch oven cool on the wire rack for some minutes and then use a plastic knife to slice the Brownie.
8. Serve and enjoy. You can serve with vanilla ice cream if you wish.

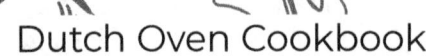

186. STRAWBERRY COBBLER

PREPARATION: 10 MIN   **COOKING:** 50 MIN   **SERVINGS:** 3

INGREDIENTS

- 3 tablespoons butter, melted
- 1 stick butter (1/2 cup), melted
- Philadelphia whipped cream cheese (8 oz.)
- 2 cans of strawberry pie filling (21 oz. Each)
- 1 box (15.25 oz.) Betty Crocker French vanilla cake mix

Nutrition: Calories 351, Fat 22g, Carbs 42g, Protein 6g

DIRECTIONS

1. Preheat your oven to 350°F.
2. Place 1/2 stick of melted butter into the bottom of a 12-inch Dutch oven. Swirl the butter around to coat the Dutch oven evenly.
3. Once done, dump both cans of strawberry pie filling inside and use a wooden spoon to spread out evenly.
4. Spread dollops of cream cheese on top of the pie filling.
5. In a bowl, mix together the remaining 1 stick of melted butter and the Cake Mix. Use a spoon or your fingers to break up the chunks.
6. Spread the mixture on top of the cream cheese dollops and pie filling.
7. Bake for 50 minutes. The top should be crispy and the edges hot and bubbly.
8. Remove and serve with vanilla ice cream if you wish.

187. BLUEBERRY DUMP CAKE

PREPARATION: 10 MIN   **COOKING:** 40 MIN   **SERVINGS:** 3

INGREDIENTS

- 1 pint blueberries
- 1/2 cup butter (1 stick, or you could use margarine)
- 1 cup milk (you can use skim or you could use almond milk or other dairy free milk in place of regular milk)
- 1 cup sugar
- 1 cup flour (all purpose or whole wheat pastry flour)

DIRECTIONS

1. Preheat your oven to 375°F and spray your Dutch oven with cooking spray or spread a bit of butter in it and set aside.
2. Melt the butter. You can melt it for 30 seconds in the microwave. In a bowl, combine the butter, flour, milk and sugar. Mix well and then pour into the prepared Dutch oven.
3. Spread the blueberries on top and then bake for 40-45 minutes. The edges should start to brown.
4. Remove from the oven and let it cool for 10 minutes. Serve.

Nutrition: Calories 372, Fat 23g, Carbs 39g, Protein 8g

188. HEAVENLY PEACH COBBLER

PREPARATION: 10 MIN **COOKING:** 20 MIN **SERVINGS:** 3

INGREDIENTS

- ½ pack vanilla cake mix
- 1 cup lemon-lime soda (Sprite/7 Up)
- 4 cups fruit (peaches, apples, berries, etc.)
- 2 tablespoons unsalted butter, cold, diced
- Whipped cream

Nutrition: Calories 282, Fat 6 g, Carbs 57g, Protein 3g

DIRECTIONS

1. Lightly grease the Dutch oven with cooking spray.
2. Add the cake mix and soda to a mixing bowl. Mix well to make a thick batter.
3. Arrange the fruit in the Dutch oven; pour the batter over it.
4. Top with the diced butter and sugar.
5. Heat the Dutch oven to 350°F.
6. Cover and cook for 20 minutes until the top is golden brown and the juices are bubbling.
7. Serve warm with whipped cream.

189. CHOCOLATE CAKE

PREPARATION: 10 MIN **COOKING:** 40 MIN **SERVINGS:** 3

INGREDIENTS

- 1 (21 oz.) can cherry pie filling
- 1 (12 oz.) can evaporate milk
- 1 regular-size pack chocolate cake mix
- ⅓ cup almonds, sliced
- ¾ cup butter, melted

Nutrition: Calories 515, Fat 24 g, Carbs 68 g, Protein 7 g

DIRECTIONS

1. Heat the Dutch oven to 350°F. Line it with parchment paper and lightly grease with cooking spray.
2. Add the pie filling and evaporated milk to a mixing bowl. Mix well.
3. Pour it over the Dutch oven and spread evenly.
4. Add the cake mix and almonds on top.
5. Drizzle the melted butter on top.
6. Cover and cook for 35–40 minutes until the cake springs back when prodded.
7. Serve warm with ice cream.

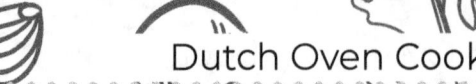

Dutch Oven Cookbook

190. CHERRY CLAFOUTI

PREPARATION: 10 MIN **COOKING:** 30 MIN **SERVINGS:** 3

INGREDIENTS

- ¾ lb. fresh or frozen and thawed cherries stemmed and pitted
- 2 large eggs
- ¼ cup of sugar
- ½ cup whole milk
- 1 teaspoon vanilla extract
- ½ cup all-purpose flour

Nutrition: Calories 92, Fat 2 g, Carbs 16 g, Protein 3 g

DIRECTIONS

1. Preheat the Dutch oven to 400°F. Evenly spread butter to cover the inside surface.
2. Spread the cherries over the bottom.
3. Whisk the eggs in a bowl. Add the sugar. Mix until well blended and frothy.
4. Add the flour, milk, and vanilla to another mixing bowl. Mix well.
5. Combine the mixtures to make a smooth batter.
6. Pour the batter over the cherries.
7. Cook, uncovered, for 30 minutes until the top is golden brown. Check by inserting a toothpick; it should come out clean. If not, cook for a few more minutes.
8. Serve warm.

191. PECAN PRALINES

PREPARATION: 10 MIN **COOKING:** 20 MIN **SERVINGS:** 3

INGREDIENTS

- 1 cup whipping cream
- 3 cups light brown sugar
- ¼ cup butter
- 2 tablespoons corn syrup
- 1 teaspoon vanilla extract

Nutrition: Calories 228, Fat 14g, Carbs 25g, Protein 2g

DIRECTIONS

1. Preheat the Dutch oven to 350°F.
2. Spread the pecan halves in the Dutch oven and cook for 5 minutes. Stir-cook for another 5 minutes. Set aside.
3. Clean the Dutch oven and add the whipping cream, brown sugar, butter, and corn syrup.
4. Boil over high heat for 4–6 minutes until the sugar melts completely, stirring occasionally.
5. Remove from heat and add the pecans and vanilla; stir for 1–2 minutes. Let cool for a while.
6. Place a spoonful of the mixture on a wax paper; allow to firm up for 10–15 minutes. Serve warm.

192. QUICK AND EASY POP BROWNIES

PREPARATION: 10 MIN   **COOKING:** 45 MIN   **SERVINGS:** 3

INGREDIENTS

- 1 box brownie mix
- 1 can soda pop
- ¾ lb. chocolate chips

Nutrition: Calories 241, Fat 13g, Carbs 35g, Protein 2g

DIRECTIONS

1. Line the Dutch oven with parchment paper.
2. Add the brownie mix and soda to a mixing bowl. Mix well until you get a smooth mixture.
3. Pour the batter over the parchment paper. Sprinkle the chocolate chips on top.
4. Heat to 350°F and bake for 45–60 minutes until well set. Check by inserting a toothpick; it should come out clean. If not, cook for a few more minutes.
5. Slice and serve warm.

193. CHOCOLATE CHIP COOKIES

PREPARATION: 10 MIN   **COOKING:** 30 MIN   **SERVINGS:** 3

INGREDIENTS

- 1 cup butter, softened
- ¾ cup packed brown sugar
- 1 egg
- 1 teaspoon baking soda
- 2¼ cups flour

Nutrition: Calories 220, Fat 11g, Carbs 29g, Protein 2g

DIRECTIONS

1. Add the butter sugar to a mixing bowl. Mix well.
2. Beat the eggs in another bowl. Mix well.
3. Add the sea salt, baking soda, and flour; mix again.
4. Combine the mixtures until smooth.
5. Divide into 24 balls.
6. Line the Dutch oven with parchment paper and lightly grease it with cooking spray.
7. Arrange the balls on the bottom.
8. Cover and cook for 6 minutes. If cookies have turned light brown, take them out. If not, cook for 2–4 more minutes. Do not overcook.
9. Let cool for a while. Serve warm.

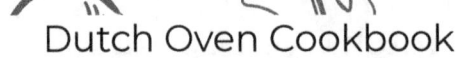

194. DUTCH OVEN BROWNIES

PREPARATION: 10 MIN **COOKING:** 40 MIN **SERVINGS:** 3

INGREDIENTS

- 1 box brownie mix
- ½ cup melted butter
- 2 large eggs
- 1 cup of chocolate chips
- 1 teaspoon vanilla extract

Nutrition: Calories 502, Fat 27g, Carbs 63.2g, Protein 5.7g

DIRECTIONS

1. Add the brownie mix to a large mixing bowl and stir in the melted butter, eggs, and water, and chocolate chips until just combined, being careful not to over-mix the batter.
2. Line the Dutch oven with a piece of parchment paper and pour in the brownie mixture.
3. Bake at 350°F for 25–30 minutes.
4. Let the brownies cool slightly and then cut into squares and serve.

195. DOUBLE CHOCOLATE CAKE

PREPARATION: 10 MIN **COOKING:** 40 MIN **SERVINGS:** 3

INGREDIENTS

- 1 box chocolate cake mix
- ¼ cup whole milk
- 1 cup of chocolate chips
- 2 cups heavy whipping cream
- 3 tablespoons powdered sugar

Nutrition: Calories 594, Fat 36.9g, Carbs 64.5g, Protein 6.3g

DIRECTIONS

1. Add the cake mix to a large mixing bowl and stir in the milk, and chocolate chips until just combined, being careful not to over-mix the batter.
2. Line the Dutch oven with a piece of parchment paper and pour in the chocolate cake mixture.
3. Bake at 350°F for about 30 minutes.
4. Remove the cake from the Dutch oven and place it on a cooling rack. Let it cool completely.
5. Add the whipping cream, powdered sugar, and vanilla extract to a large mixing bowl and beat with a hand mixer.
6. Cut the chocolate cake in half to create two layers. Spread half of the whipped cream on one layer, cover with the second layer and decorate the whole cake with whipped cream.
7. If desired, sprinkle with more chocolate chips for better presentation.

196. VERRY BERRY SWIRL

PREPARATION: 10 MIN **COOKING:** 40 MIN **SERVINGS:** 3

INGREDIENTS

- 1 (14 oz.) pizza dough
- 3 cups frozen or fresh mixed berries
- ¾ cup granulated sugar
- ½ teaspoon cinnamon
- 2 tablespoons all-purpose flour

Nutrition: Calories 473, Fat 20.7g, Carbs 68.6g, Protein 4.6g

DIRECTIONS

1. Roll out the pizza dough into a ¼-inch-thick square.
2. Sprinkle the mixed berries, granulated sugar, cinnamon, and all-purpose flour on top. Ensure that every berry is coated with flour so that a nice thick sauce will form during baking.
3. Roll up the dough with the berries inside and cut diagonally with a sharp knife.
4. Carefully twist both parts of the dough together to make one long braid.
5. Shape the braid into a circle and place it in the Dutch oven on top of a parchment paper piece.
6. Bake at 350°F for 30–40 minutes.
7. Let cool slightly and then dust with powdered sugar when ready to serve.

197. PEACH COBBLER

PREPARATION: 10 MIN **COOKING:** 30 MIN **SERVINGS:** 3

INGREDIENTS

- 2 tablespoons butter
- 1 cup sugar (divided)
- 1 cup all-purpose flour
- 1 tablespoon baking powder
- ½ cup whole milk

Nutrition: Calories 615, Fat 25g, Carbs 58g, Protein 6.6g

DIRECTIONS

1. Grease the Dutch oven well on every side with the two tablespoons of butter.
2. Arrange the peach slices in the Dutch oven and sprinkle with ¾ cup of the sugar.
3. Add the flour, baking powder, melted butter, milk, and remaining sugar to a bowl.
4. Mix until combined and then use an ice cream scoop to deposit the batter on top of the peaches in the Dutch oven.
5. Bake at 350°F for 30–35 minutes.
6. Let cool slightly and then dust with powdered sugar when ready to serve.

Dutch Oven Cookbook

198. APPLE CRISP

PREPARATION: 10 MIN **COOKING:** 40 MIN **SERVINGS:** 3

INGREDIENTS

- 6 apples, cored and cut into wedges
- 1 cup all-purpose flour
- ½ cup of sugar
- ¾ cup butter
- 1 teaspoon cinnamon

Nutrition: Calories 459, Fat 23.6g, Carbs 43.7g, Protein 3g

DIRECTIONS

1. Grease the Dutch oven and place the apple wedges in the bottom.
2. Pour in the water and let sit for 5 minutes.
3. Meanwhile, blend the flour, sugar, butter, and cinnamon in a food processor until a crumbly dough forms.
4. Distribute the dough on top of the apples, making sure you fill every hole, and bake, covered, for about 25 minutes at 350°F.
5. Remove the lid and cook uncovered for another 10–15 minutes until golden brown.
6. Serve warm with a scoop of ice cream.

199. ALL IN ONE APPLE CAKE

PREPARATION: 10 MIN **COOKING:** 40 MIN **SERVINGS:** 3

INGREDIENTS

- 3 apples, cored and cut into wedges
- ½ cup butter softened
- ½ cup of sugar, 2 large eggs
- 1¼ cups self-rising flour
- ½ cup whole milk

Nutrition: Calories 290, Fat 13.6g, Carbs 39.8g, Protein 4.4g

DIRECTIONS

1. Grease the Dutch oven with a small piece of butter.
2. Add the butter and the sugar to a large mixing bowl and beat with a hand mixer until fluffy.
3. Stir in the eggs one at a time, mixing well after each addition.
4. Stir in the flour and mix until just combined.
5. Stir in the apple wedges and mix with a spatula.
6. Pour the cake mixture into the buttered Dutch oven and bake at 350°F about 40 minutes.
7. Let the cake cool slightly before serving with a sprinkle of powdered sugar.

200. DUTCH OVEN CHOCOLATE CHIP COOKIES

PREPARATION: 10 MIN **COOKING:** 20 MIN **SERVINGS:** 3

INGREDIENTS

- ½ cup butter, melted
- ¾ cup light brown sugar
- 2 teaspoons vanilla extract
- 2 large eggs, room temperature
- 1½ cups self-rising flour

Nutrition: Calories 496, Fat 25.6g, Carbs 58.6g, Protein 7.7g

DIRECTIONS

1. Grease the Dutch oven with a little bit of butter.
2. Add the melted butter, sugar, vanilla extract, and eggs to a large mixing bowl.
3. Mix until combined and stir in the flour.
4. Mix in the chocolate chips and transfer the cookie dough to the buttered Dutch oven.
5. Bake at 350°F for about 20 minutes.

CONCLUSION

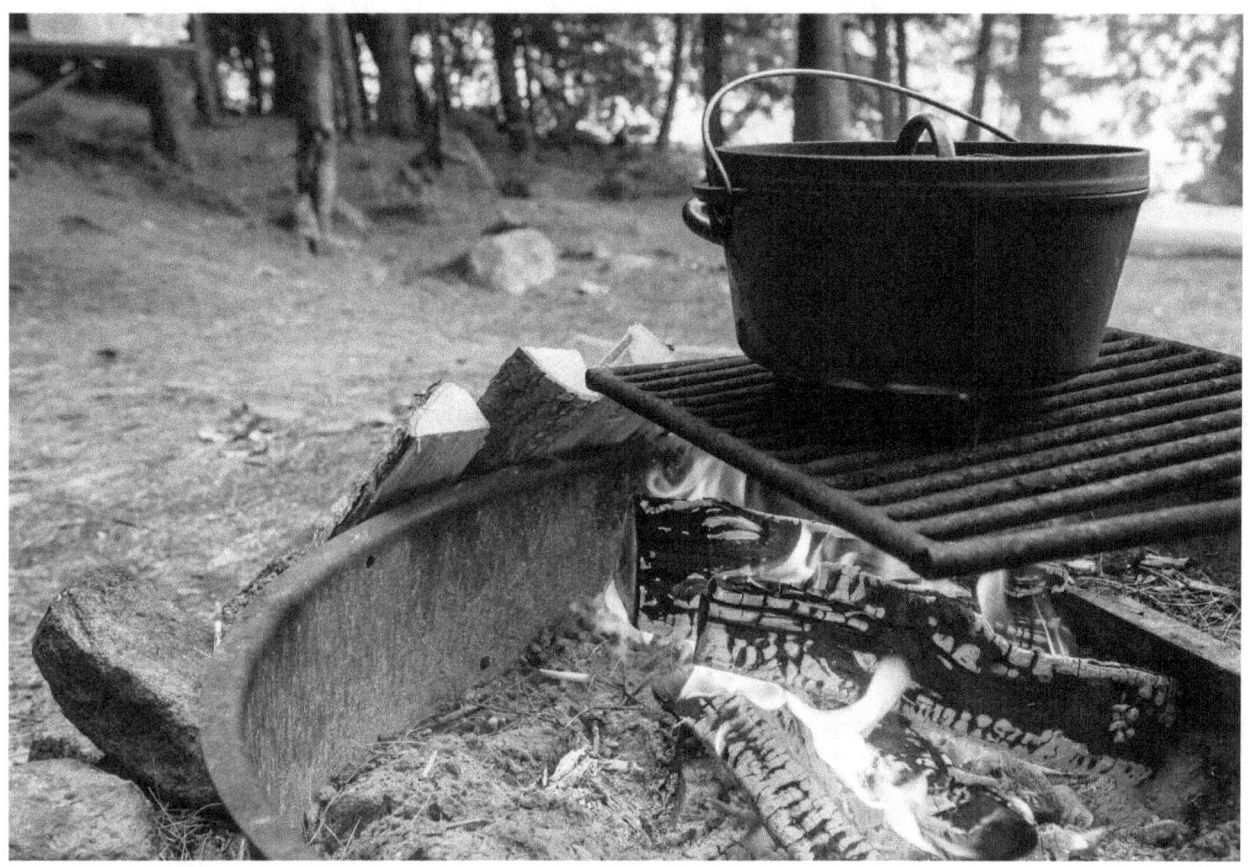

Once you try some of the foods in this book, you will see how simple and enjoyable it is to incorporate the 5-ingredient meals into your life on a regular basis, especially with the help of a Dutch oven. The dishes in this book range from simple to elegant, and there is something for all tastes and occasions. You have now begun your introduction to the simplified and delicious world of limited cooking ingredients with a Dutch oven. Gone are the days of avoiding the kitchen because you were afraid of getting stuck in it all day.

Now that you are familiar with the Dutch oven techniques and 5-ingredient cooking, you can take the next step and get more creative. Create your own recipes with an open mind when shopping for food. Let your gastronomic instincts be guided by the seasons. When you tune into the natural characteristics and flavors of healthy ingredients, you will find that the ingredients seem to fit together, and you can instinctively create quick and tasty meals. The simplest meals are usually the most delicious, not only because they bring out pure flavors, but also because of the enjoyment you experience during their creation.

Cooking with fewer ingredients isn't new, but it's a smart choice that lets you recreate the magic of complex and time-consuming kitchens with less effort by tossing the right mix of ingredients into your Dutch oven. When you have only a few ingredients to use, you can design ahead and fill your closet in advance with these essential ingredients. When most of

Dutch Oven Cookbook

your ingredients are on the shelf and waiting to be added, it makes cooking extremely smooth and easy.

When you're stuck in the daily collection of relaxation, electronics, and commitments, camping is a great haven. It is very healing to get out into nature and breathe in some fresh air.

With this book, we hope you take that outdoor enjoyment to the next level, with easy meals prepared over a fire or charcoal in the field. If your kids haven't experienced the joy of a simple, nutritious meal with little grass or twigs, now is the time to get out there. There is something here for the wealthiest diners and you won't regret trying the outdoor cooking!
I hope the book has opened your eyes to the endless ways you can make simple 5-ingredient meals with your Dutch oven. Now it is your turn to act. Get started preparing as many recipes we've talked about as possible to get the most out of your Dutch oven!

Dutch Oven Cookbook

RECIPES INDEX

INTRODUCTION 5
WHAT YOU NEED TO KNOW
ABOUT DUTCH OVENS 7

BREAKFAST 13
1. Campfire Breakfast 14
2. Yummy Cobbler 14
3. Pancakes 15
4. Dutch Oven Scrambled Eggs and Biscuits Recipe 15
5. Eggs Benedict Casserole 16
6. Dutch Oven Eggs Baked in Avocados 16
7. Camp Quiche 16
8. Australian Damper 17
9. Country Breakfast 17
10. Breakfast Omelet 18
11. Crab & fennel spaghetti 18
12. Epic rib-eye steak 19
13. Quinoa, Everyday Dals, And Avocado 19
14. Easy sausage carbonara 20
15. Brown Rice, Everyday Dals, & Avocado 20
16. Dutch Camping Farmers' Breakfast 21

POULTRY 22
17. Classic Chicken "Stir Fry" 23
18. Balsamic Vinegar Chicken 23
19. Chicken Over the Coals 23
20. Chicken Kebabs 24
21. Chicken and Potatoes 24
22. Creamy Santa Fe Chicken 24
23. Mediterranean Chicken 25
24. Rosemary Chicken Bake 25
25. Chicken with Cornbread Stuffing 26
26. Leek and Dijon Chicken 26
27. Asian BBQ Chicken 27
28. Chicken Piccata 27
29. Sweet chicken surprise 28
30. Thai red chicken soup 28
31. Chicken in a Pot 29
32. Easy Chicken Dinner 29
33. Easy Chicken Casserole 30
34. Scrambled egg omelette 30

Vegetarian and Side Dish Recipes 31
35. Dutch Potato and Egg Scramble 32
36. Dutch Oven Mountain Man 32
37. Dutch over Potatoes with Cheese 33
38. Dutch Oven Ravioli 33
39. Grilled Sweet Potato Fries 34
40. Blistered Shishito Peppers 34
41. Bubble and Squeak 35
42. Sizzling seared scallops 35
43. Pan Toasted Couscous 36
44. Fresh Cucumber Salad 36
45. Sweet Roasted Root Vegetables 37
46. Fennel Gratin 37
47. Buttered Corn and Poblano Soup 38
48. Pita Pizza Blanco 38
49. Ancient Grain Stuffed Peppers 39
50. Parmesan Risotto 39
51. All-Time Favorite Mac and Cheese 40
52. Creamy Mushroom Pasta 40
53. Mascarpone Pumpkin Pasta 41
54. Classic Cheesy Spaghetti 41
55. Braised Leeks 42
56. French Onion Pasta 42
57. Seasoned French Fries 43
58. Buttery Carrots 43
59. Baked Garlic and Mushroom Rice 44
60. Quinoa with Mixed Vegetables and Artichoke Hearts 44
61. Dutch Oven Vegetarian Lasagna 45
62. Cheesy Ravioli Pasta Bake 45
63. Vegetarian Jambalaya 46
64. Stuffed Zucchini 46

Soup and Stew 47
65. Vegetable Stew 48
66. Stuffed Bell Peppers 48
67. Sausage, Pepper & Potato Packets 49
68. Chicken Mushroom Soup 49
69. Creme Potato Chicken Soup 50
70. Beef and Cabbage Soup 50
71. Quinoa Chickpea Corn Soup 51
72. Sweet Potato Soup 51
73. Pork and Bean Soup 51
74. Tomato Cream Soup with Basil 52
75. Chicken Bean Barley Soup 52
76. Collard Green White Bean Soup with Sausages 53
77. Bacon and Potato Soup 53
78. Vegetable Soup 54
79. Jerusalem Artichoke Soup 54
80. Black Bean Soup 55
81. Corn and Black Bean Soup 55
82. Potato Soup 56
83. Cauliflower Soup 56
84. Miso Soup 57
85. Tomato Tortellini Soup 57
86. Broccoli Cheese Soup 57

Fish and Seafood Recipes 58
87. Tilapia with Chive Blessing 59
88. Pasta with Clams and Pancetta 59
89. Beer Mustard Shrimp 60
90. Tilapia Nuggets 60
91. Baked Salmon with Herbs 60
92. Baked Trout with Cherry Tomatoes 61
93. Tilapia Cacciatore 61
94. Seafood Risotto 62
95. Calamari Fra Diavolo 62
96. Seafood Stew 63
97. Cajun Scallops 63
98. Sort of salmon niçoise 64
99. Seared Salmon with Caper Sauce 64
100. Foil Pack Grilled Lemony Salmon with Asparagus 65
101. Creamy Herbed Shrimp Pasta 65

102. Kissed by an Italian Whitefish	66
103. Fresh and Simple Fish Tacos	66
104. Lemon Shrimp and Pasta	66
105. Lemon Butter Salmon Foil Packs	67
106. Fish Tacos	67
107. Foil Packed Honey-Lime Tilapia and Corn	67
108. Cilantro-Lime Shrimp Foil Packs	68
109. Fish and Vegetables on a Skewer	68
110. Garlic Shrimp	68
111. Dutch Oven-baked Salmon	69
112. Beer Me-Lightly Fried Fish Fillets	69
BEEF	**70**
113. Italian seared beef	71
114. Ground Beef Skewers	71
115. Beef & Potato Packets	72
116. Ann's Brisket	72
117. Swiss Steak	72
118. Onion Swiss Steak	73
119. Poor Man's Steak	73
120. Corned Beef & Cabbage	73
121. Sausage Balls	74
122. Great Beef Stew	74
123. Beef Goulash	74
124. Mess	75
125. Taco Pie	75
126. Bacon, Beef, And Beans Casserole	75
127. Spinach Steak Pinwheels	76
128. Sunday Roast Beef and Gravy	76
129. Beef and Vegetable Stir Fry	77
130. Balsamic Braised Beef Ribs	77
131. Grandma's Weekend Roast	78
132. Flank Steak Roulade	78
133. Jalapeño Beef Pouches	79
134. Steak and Crispy Beet Salad	79
135. Ginger Spiced Beef	80
Pork and Lamb Recipes	81
136. Roast Pork with Blueberry Sauce	82
137. Smokey Carbonara	82
138. Overstuffed Pork Chops	83
139. Parmesan Polenta with Crispy Prosciutto	83
140. Pancetta and Asparagus Linguine	84
141. Slow Cooker Pulled Pork	84
142. Stuffed Pork Sausage	85
143. Lovely lamb hotpots	85
144. Smoky Split Pea Soup with Bacon	86
145. Creamy Tortellini with Peas and Crispy Prosciutto	86
146. Sweet and Sticky Pork Chops	87
147. New England Ham Boil	87
148. Italian Roast Pork	88
149. Country-Style Pork Ragù	88
150. Beer Brats with Sauerkraut	89
151. Sausage and Peppers with Blistered Cherry Tomatoes	89
152. Smoked Sausage and White Bean Cassoulet	90
153. Seared Lamb Chops with Lemon and Oregano	90
154. Irish Pub Lamb Stew	91
155. Garlic and Rosemary Roasted Leg of Lamb	91
BREAD, ROLLS AND BISCUITS.	**92**
156. Jalapeno Dutch oven Crusty Bread	93
157. Dutch Oven Cobbler	93
158. Lemony courgette linguine	94
159. Dutch oven Campfire Biscuits	94
160. Pizza Pie in a Dutch oven	95
161. Dutch Oven Pizza	95
162. Double Baked Potato Boat	96
163. Cheat Doughnuts	96
164. Rustic Bread	97
165. Dutch Oven Monkey Bread with Cinnamon	98
166. Dutch Oven Rolls	98
167. No-Knead Bread	99
168. Breakfast Cinnamon Rolls	99
169. Almond pastry puff	100
170. Speedy steamed pudding pots	100
171. Egg & mango chutney flatbreads	101
DESSERT RECIPES	**102**
172. Honeyed Figs and Ricotta	103
173. Wildberry Mascarpone Sliders	103
174. Coconut Mandarin Cake	104
175. Gingered Chocolate Bark	104
176. Rich Brioche Pudding	105
177. Baked Apples With Buttered Pecans	105
178. Granola Over A Campfire	106
179. Cheesecake Dutch oven Recipe	106
180. Corn and Corn Fritters	107
181. Bacon and Cheddar Cheese	107
182. 1 Pot Fettuccine Alfredo Recipe	108
183. Chocolate Butterfinger Cake	108
184. Apple Dump Cake	109
185. Dutch Oven Brownie	109
186. Strawberry Cobbler	110
187. Blueberry Dump Cake	110
188. Heavenly Peach Cobbler	111
189. Chocolate Cake	111
190. Cherry Clafouti	112
191. Pecan Pralines	112
192. Quick and Easy Pop Brownies	113
193. Chocolate Chip Cookies	113
194. Dutch Oven Brownies	114
195. Double Chocolate Cake	114
196. Verry Berry Swirl	115
197. Peach Cobbler	115
198. Apple Crisp	116
199. All in One Apple Cake	116
200. Dutch Oven Chocolate Chip Cookies	116
CONCLUSION	**117**

www.ingramcontent.com/pod-product-compliance
Lightning Source LLC
Chambersburg PA
CBHW080458240426
43673CB00005B/234